Still Lives

Still Lives

Narratives of Spinal Cord Injury

Jonathan Cole

A Bradford Book
The MIT Press
Cambridge, Massachusetts
London, England

This book was set in Sabon and Meta by Achorn Graphic Services, Inc. Printed and bound in the United States of America.

Library of Congress Cataloging-in-Publication Data

Cole, Jonathan (Jonathan David)
  Still lives : narratives of spinal cord injury / Jonathan Cole.
    p. cm.
  Includes bibliographical references and index.
  ISBN 0-262-03315-1 (alk. paper)
  1. Quadriplegics—Great Britain—Biography. I. Title.
RC406.Q33C64   2004
362.4'3'092241—dc22

                                        2003059378

10 9 8 7 6 5 4 3 2 1

For my mother

To my wife, Sue, and our daughters (in order of appearance): Eleanor, Lydia, Celia, and Georgia.

Contents

Acknowledgments

I am most grateful to those who invited me, a stranger, into their homes and offices. They allowed me to sit and listen as they discussed their, or their partner's, spinal cord injury and its consequences, and then trusted me to write what I could. These twelve narratives form the heart of this book.

In the course of researching the book I spoke with several medical and paramedical workers, and I thank all who gave their time to listen to my unformed and sometimes naïve thoughts. Thanks are due to Tony Tromans, Anne Seaman, Nigel North, and members of the physiotherapy and occupational therapy departments in the Duke of Cornwall Spinal Treatment Centre, Salisbury. My secretary Sharon Evans also helped by transcribing some of the interviews.

These days it is not easy to find people able to talk about their experiences; medical records are confidential and out of bounds. In any case, I did not want to go to patients as a doctor and so would have spurned a medical route. I am very grateful to the various contacts and friends who suggested people I might go to see. In this I must mention Nigel North and Stephen Duckworth for their assistance, and the Spinal Injuries Association for kindly agreeing to run a small piece inviting people to contact me. In the end, I had more volunteers than I could possibly see; my thanks and apologies are due to those I could not visit and to those I saw but whose stories are not within this book.

I was fortunate that Nigel North, Max Bowker, and Jan Smart volunteered to read the manuscript and satisfied me as to its tone, with Max ending up a brilliant proofreader, too.

To write a book is an enormous privilege. I must thank Barbara Murphy and Sara Meirowitz, and before them Michael Rutter, for commissioning me to write something once more and then agreeing to the subject, and for their support during the long process itself. Barbara and Sara and then Katherine Almeida also guided my draft to completed manuscript with a beautiful combination of enthusiasm, lightness, and thoroughness.

Chekhov once famously gave advice to a young writer, along the lines of "Get a day job." My day job is as a full-time clinical neurophysiologist in several hospitals. I juggle this with some academic research, too, so life is quite busy. Writing may be a solitary occupation, but the process can only be done with the support and assistance of those round about. My wife, Sue, has been in the background throughout, enabling my hours of writing and travels to meet people, as she maintained the threads of our life. Similarly, our daughters have watched me disappear into the study uncomplainingly. So it is to them that this book should, and must, be dedicated.

Science manipulates things and gives up living in them.

—Maurice Merleau-Ponty, 1964. From "Eye and Mind," in *The Primacy of Perception*

The promise of art and revolution is that people might discard their preconceptions and truly understand what it is in the mind of another. What would the world look like in which people dare to wish to know what it is like not to walk?

—John Hockenberry, 1995. *Moving Violations*

Nothing is more difficult than facing concepts *without prejudice.*

—Ludwig Wittgenstein, 1980. *Remarks on the Philosophy of Psychology*

Introduction

1 Twenty Years On

A Lost Beginning

A little under twenty years ago, I was a research fellow trying to use a neurophysiological technique, spinal cord stimulation, for the relief of chronic pain in those with spinal cord injury. I spent lots of time with patients, during their visits to the hospital, in their homes, and even in pubs where we could sit and chat without the doctor/patient thing in the way. They would bemoan their pain and the poor treatment of it. Many had given up discussing pain with doctors, since conventional medicine had so little to offer. Some had tried aspirin, others morphine; a few found alcohol so useful they were concerned about addiction. Their proper doctors had little time to listen; some did not even accept their levels of pain.

My research project only showed the treatment to be ineffective in most pains. Indeed, in the end, and not before time, I realized that my project could never work, because for sound physiological principles it was inappropriate.[1, 2]

The people I tried to help were philosophical; they had lost nothing. But I felt I had let them down. I had not been able to relieve the pain after raising their hopes. Nor was I sure I had really understood their condition.

Action Man

Some years later, I was lecturing at a meeting in London. The applause seemed genuine, and the questions interested rather than simply polite. I could relax as I listened to the next speaker and look forward to supper. After all, The Royal Society of Medicine did a reasonable spread. It was a joint meeting of the neurology and rehabilitation sections, and the next lecturer was from Dublin, speaking on spinal cord injury. Nothing new there, I thought.

He began with a video of a man with a high tetraplegia, with no movement or feeling below the neck, competing in a paraplegic games. Unable to move much more than his neck and face, the man had a crossbow mounted in front of him. He controlled its direction and elevation through a small mouth-organ device connected to the bow by a motor. He'd puff at one end, and the bow moved down; a puff or suck the other and it turned to the right or left. The film seemed old, and the man had the cropped hair, square-jawed look of a serviceman after the war. Slowly and with evident deliberation, he took aim, calculating the wind strength and the necessary elevation and direction, before he puffed into the center of the mouthpiece and shot the arrow.

I never saw if the arrow hit the target, and I remember little of the lecture. I sat there fascinated by the short film and by the way the man had interacted with the world. Though almost immobile, he had imposed his will and made an action—via the small mouthpiece—to unleash the arrow. He would have seen the hit and been delighted or frustrated by his aim, just as I would have, even if his body's involvement was reduced to his airway and lips, whereas I would have been standing, bow pulled back, arm outstretched, trigger fingers poised, eye in line, my whole body within the action.

In the second or so when he had broken his neck, that man had been transformed from a man of action, as a soldier or a lad about town, immersed in physical challenges, to an intellectual, able to exercise his mind and move a few facial, head, and neck muscles. The man, possibly a soldier, would have scoffed, "Me, an intellectual? Forget it." Yet, almost perversely, it seemed true. What he had previously done with his body, without a thought, was now beyond him. What he could do now he had to think about deliberately and in new ways. How had he coped with the change, and how did he feel?

Most of us pay little attention to our bodies. They are usually absent from our awareness, just allowing us to do what we like. We walk, talk, sit, and write with no conscious attention to these acts. Our bodies are our instruments, the mechanisms of their functioning automated, and beyond our will or conscious attention. After spinal cord injury, the body is absented, insentient and unmoving, and yet has to be looked after, because it no longer functions automatically. People, I presumed, have to attend to their bodies in a wholly new way. Robert Murphy, in his moving and profound account of becoming tetraplegic, interestingly called *The Body Silent,* described this: "my former sense of embodiment remained taken for granted . . . my [new] sense of re-embodiment is problematic negative and conscious. . . . Consuming consciousness of handicap even invades one's dreams."[3]

Again and again, as we shall see, for tetraplegics, what previously took care of itself has to be known and looked after consciously, intellectually, and remorselessly, whether it is skin pressure care, bladder emptying, or bowel care, because those functions are no longer connected with their command centers in the brain stem. Those with spinal cord injury are condemned to an intellectual interest in their bodies in order to continue their lives.

At another level, we are aware of our bodies and take pleasure from our body, in exercise or a bath, or even during sex. We also have a conscious sense of our appearance, seen in our relations with others and in developing our self-esteem. What we look like and how we move, as well as what we say, play a large part in how we are perceived. In our emotional lives, as Merleau-Ponty wrote, "the body is more than a means, it is our expression in the world."[4] For those with spinal cord injury, their bodies and hence their worlds might change. How?

In his famous essay "The Disembodied Lady," about a person who had lost all sensations of movement and position sense from below the face area, Oliver Sacks described how, initially unable to control movements, she felt less "in her body."[5] GL, with a similar but worse condition (she has lost cutaneous sensation as well as movement and position sense from the lower face down), has described how she feels like a pilot of her body rather than in it. Her "deafferentation" is from the lower face, and she has to think to control her head and neck movements, a huge additional task. I have written about a subject and friend, Ian Waterman, with a similar loss of movement and position sense, and cutaneous touch below the neck.[6] He has normal neck sensation, and after an initial period of being unable to control any movement, has learned over years to stand and walk and to live independently. Ian does not consider himself disembodied—he is in and of his body. Interestingly, both he and GL have invested much time not simply in relearning locomotor and instrumental action, but also in relearning gesture. It was important for them to be emotionally expressive in their bodies.

Though Ian does not dwell on the time of his illness—it was more than thirty years ago now and a terrible time for him—it is clear that when, initially, he was lying on his bed and was completely unable to control movement in any way, he felt most disembodied. Ian described how, as he began to realize that he could control movement through thought and "visual supervision," he began to feel more at home with his body. His re-embodiment seemed to require both a sense of making the movement and seeing that movement made successfully. In other words, a sense of agency or will,[7] as well as feedback of movement, seem necessary to feel at one with one's body.

What, I wondered, did the man with the crossbow feel about his body? If sensation is reduced or even taken away from much of the body, and if movement, likewise, almost impossible, then he was reduced largely to observing. How might he view his body? More as an object and as a thing—if so, then where did he reside? Without movement, without gesture, without independence of action in the world, what was left of will? In his account of his own descent into tetraplegia, Robert Murphy wrote of the alterations that occurred in his will, even associated with a relatively simple movement: "For a while I tried to will the legs to move, but each futile attempt was psychologically devastating. . . . I was saved from the edge of breakdown because the slow process of paralysis of my limbs was paralleled by a progressive atrophy of the need and impulse for physical activity. I was losing the will to move."[8]

The injury had altered his relation to his body and to others in huge and unimagined ways, from knowledge of his body to his will to move and his psychological integrity.

An Arm Full of Pepper

For some time I had wondered about the pain that those with spinal cord injury complained of. How might that affect someone with no movement or sensation? Then I had a short burst of severe pain during a research visit to Germany.

We had arrived on the overnight train from Munich, groggy from a sleepless journey and still unsure why we had been woken for breakfast on the train at 5 a.m., leaving us two miserable hours of semi-wakefulness, watching a cold dawn light the snowy countryside. Rolf-Detlef introduced himself to us at Hamburg station and took us to his lab. Though still bewildered, we accepted his offer of another breakfast before he showed us around. It was clear that he was proudest of the laser used in some experiments on the perception and transmission of pain; in the wrong hands, he told me, it could cut through metal.

I was the first to do the experiment. Rolf-Detlef led me into a windowless room, where I sat facing a wall, with a low table in front of me. He explained that the pain would last sixteen minutes and I was to let him know its severity each minute. Then I felt a pinprick in the forearm as he injected the dose of pepper extract. Despite my preparation for the shock—let alone my desire not to put off my colleague, Ian, who was next in line—the pain made me gasp. My body hunched and my neck dropped. Ian saw despite my silence.

But I was not aware of all this; I could think of little but the pain. When the chemical went in I was aware of a short flush of warmth and then, almost immediately, came the pain. Television or movies sometimes show explosions as tiny areas of bright light that expand to fill the whole screen, destroying size and context and perspective as the screen fills. Similarly, my pain was difficult to localize; it was out there and below me, though I was no longer sure quite what that meant. It filled my arm, my body, and my sense of self. Pain destroyed my perspective and even my perception of me.

I had lived until then with a perception of my body as a whole. Even when not attending to it, I knew of and felt a presence of body, of an arm or a leg. But with the pain, I no longer thought in such terms. I had a pain that intellectually I knew was out there, but it took over so much that further localization was impossible. More than that, however, I no longer had a background thought of my hand or arm at all. In an existential way, the pain removed my feeling of being embodied: I just had pain. My perception of a shaped arm and hand was absent, overwhelmed and driven from me by the pain. I could think of nothing. I may have slumped, I did not know; I just knew pain, pain filled my body and my self, with no room for other thoughts or feelings. I tried to explore and to analyze, but its grip was too great. I just existed, though quite what "I" was, I no longer knew; it was a me-with-pain, no longer an "I," no longer a self observing the world or even immersed in it, for my immersion in the pain was so consuming that the world, as an external place to calibrate myself in, and from, no longer presented itself to me.

After a minute (was that all?), Rolf-Detlef called out for my pain rating. "Severe." I shouted the same again a minute later. After that, thankfully, it peaked and I began to view the world and myself in it again. I could even observe the pain as it ebbed, rather than just exist with it. As my ratings of its severity subsided, I rejoined the others in the room, in the world. After twelve minutes or so, the pain was gone and I could joke about the "minor irritation" Ian was about to enjoy.

Ian did the experiment. I could see his discomfort and could empathize with him, with a matchless intensity and immediacy. Then Ian returned to our world and we broke for coffee. Some experiments, we agreed, are more fun than others.[9]

We went on to other experiments, and the pain faded from our view and memory.[10] That night, tired from a sleepless night and a busy day, Ian and I had supper together. We talked of much, but neither of us thought it worthwhile mentioning the pain. It was safely in the past, just another experiment. Yet over the next few days, I could not help but think about my pain; I had had a few minutes of experimentally induced severe pain, which I had known would soon be over. But what, I wondered, of the patients I had seen over the years with pain of varying intensities and durations? How inadequate had my response to them been? I had seen how little Ian's expression communicated his pain. I would have had little idea of his experience if I had not just shared it myself. What of patients? How had they endured and communicated their pains? How had pain imposed on their lives?

Nothing to Say

When I thought about my pain, I described the effect that it had on me but had no words for the experience itself. Are there no words for what pain is like that describe it exactly? Arthur Frank in describing, or attempting to explain his own pain, wrote:

We have plenty of words to describe specific pains: sharp, throbbing, piercing, burning, even dull. But these words do not describe the experience of pain. We lack terms to express what it means to live "in" such pain. Unable to express pain, we come to believe there is *nothing to say* [my italics]. Like a sick feeling that comes with the recognition of yourself as ill, there is a pain attached to being in pain.[11]

If pain was so difficult to express, even when we had all shared something of the experience, what of the numbness and lack of sensation of those with spinal cord injury? Were there no words for that, either?

I went to talk with a friend who works in a spinal cord injury center. I said I would like to sit with people with cord injuries to ask them how they cope and how they have learned new ways of living. I could see by his body language that there was a problem. Medical staff, he said, try not to get too deep, for that might lead to patients being confronted with something they could not face. I agreed that it might only be possible with those aware of my aim and strong enough to go the distance. But maybe many were. Robert Murphy had commented on this too: "Nobody has ever asked me what it is like to be a paraplegic—and now a quadriplegic— for this would violate all the rules of middle class etiquette."[12]

I respected the feelings of those who worked with patients, but not convinced by my friend's advice. After all, to live with spinal cord injury could not be done without, at some time, confronting it and coming to an accommodation with it. Chronic pain could not be ignored either. If not discussed with medical staff, then it would have to be with friends and family. I wanted to violate a few rules to try to understand. This is not to say that there have not been books on both conditions, and many fine ones, including Christopher Reeve's, full of modesty and resolve.[13] But my aim was to look at a range of experiences of living with spinal cord injury, from soon after to years later, to understand what it was like.

It seemed a propitious time. Spinal cord injury medicine has not historically been in the forefront of neurological research. In the United

Kingdom, the hospitals for those with cord injuries have been sited well away from mainstream neurology wards and medical schools, in backwaters, hidden—until recently—from both public gaze and, alas, grant-giving bodies. That the situation is now changing is due both to the resourcefulness of those with cord injuries and to the fact that now, steadily, scientists are making important discoveries that may lead to new treatments.

The use of external neural stimulation of muscles, or nerve roots, or even the spinal cord may allow for far greater movement than people with spinal cord injury have previously had. At a more fundamental level, the old dictum that the adult nervous system is capable of little recovery once damaged may need to be revised, and several projects are underway to try to help patients recover function lost after spinal injury. The discovery of various nerve growth factors allows us to consider whether nerve roots may grow back into the spinal cord after injury and, after that, if the major pathways in the spinal cord may be helped to regenerate. Perhaps this is a false dawn, but it is nevertheless the first real dawn that the spinal cord injured community have had for some considerable time.

The fact remains, however, that for most people with spinal cord injury their problems have been present for many years and may well, unfortunately, persist for years, too. At one level, I was concerned to understand what it is like to exist with these conditions, and what sort of lives these people create with—and despite—their profound problems.

There have been many books involving neurological case studies; these neurological mishaps can certainly illuminate something of what it is to be human. Often such stories focus on the obscure and bizarre: losses of balance, or of sensation, neglect of part of one's body, blindsight, and prosopagnosia. I am no less guilty than anyone else: I have written a book about a condition with fewer than ten known cases, and am happy to defend this.[14] Because of the fantastic nature of some conditions, a reviewer of one of Oliver Sacks' books went so far as to write that neurologists seem to have all the good stories. But more prosaic and common conditions such as spinal cord injury have much to teach us, if only we listen and look long enough. These stories are not appealing because the conditions are extraordinary or rare but because they reveal the responses of ordinary people to them.

The Physical Loss

No narrative of living with a spinal cord injury can be complete without some knowledge of the physical changes that occur as a result of the injury (see figures 1.1 and 1.2 and table 1.1).

The spinal cord begins at the neck and extends down to the low back, supported and protected by the vertebral column. The sensory nerves leave the cord and the motor, or movement, ones enter it through nerve roots at each vertebral level. These levels are broadly divided into the neck, or cervical (with eight vertebrae and eight root levels); chest, or thoracic

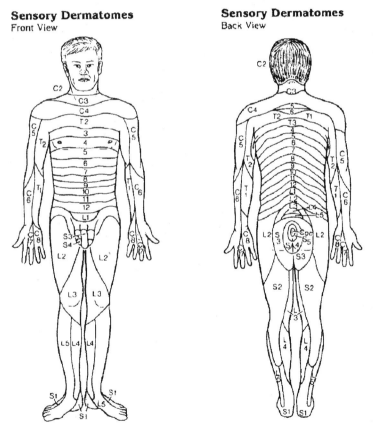

Sensory Dermatomes
Front View

Sensory Dermatomes
Back View

Figure 1.1
Sensory levels; areas of skin supplied by each spinal root. (1989 Standards of the American Spinal Injuries Association. Reproduced by permission of the American Spinal Injury Association, Chicago, IL.)

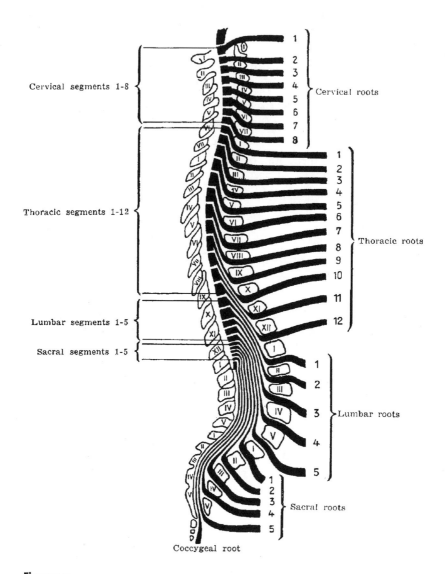

Figure 1.2

The relation between spinal cord segment, vertebral column level, and spinal nerve root nomenclature. (Reproduced by permission from Guttmann, Sir Ludwig, 1973. Spinal Cord Injuries. Comprehensive management and research. Oxford: Blackwell.)

Table 1.1
The relation between spinal nerve root level and various movements

Movement	Spinal root level
Diaphragm	C3 C4 C5
Shoulder out	C5 C6
Elbow bending	C5 C6
Elbow straightening	C6 C7 C8
Wrist bending	C6 C7
Wrist straightening	C7 C8
Finger straightening	C7 C8
Finger bending	C7 C8 T1
Hand muscles	C8 T1
Hip bending	L1 L2 L3
Knee straightening	L3 L4
Hip straightening	L4 L5 S1
Foot lifting	L4 L5 S1
Foot pointing	S1 S2
Toe movement	L5 S1 S2

Note that each movement is dependent on more than one root and that most roots contribute to more than one movement.

(twelve roots); low back, or lumbar (five roots); and pelvic area, or sacral (five roots). The level of an injury is described in terms of its root level, with a high cervical injury being, say, C3, and a low back one L5. An injury in the cervical area will lead to loss of use of arms, trunk, and legs, a tetraplegia if complete, or a tetraparesis if some movement remains. Injury to the thoracic, lumbar, and sacral cord leads to loss of movement of the legs but spares the arms—paraplegia if complete, and paraparesis if incomplete.

Any spinal cord injury may be temporary or permanent. Most injuries involve some initial swelling as well as more serious damage, so some recovery may occur, which is one reason why prognosis can initially be difficult. Because the cord is arranged, in cross section, with nerve fibers involved in touch and movement sensation in its upper half and those fibers involved in movement and pain and temperature sensation in the lower half, it is possible to have a cord syndrome with loss of movement and pain/temperature sensory loss but some touch sensation remaining, or one in which movement remains but touch and movement and position sense are lost. Usually, though, the impairment is not so neat as this, and some or all of both are affected to varying amounts.

The functions of the cord are reflected in the neurological impairments following damage to it. These may be divided into movement or motor function, to voluntary muscles as well as to the breathing system, gut, bladder, and blood vessels, and sensory function to skin, muscles, and internal organs. Because different sensory and motor nerves pass in and out at each level and because the cord is the relay of fibers to and from the brain, the level of injury is crucial.

Those injured at C1 and C2 will have no movement and sensation below the head. They will be dependent on a respirator because the nerves controlling breathing exit at C3. C3 tetraplegics may be able to control an electric wheelchair via a head control, but will still need assistance with breathing. Someone with a C4 level may be able to breathe unaided using the diaphragm, though he or she (and anyone with an level above T8 or so) will still have lost chest wall movement and have reduced expansion of the lungs. A C5 lesion will allow some movement of the shoulders and of biceps, allowing elbow flexion, but no power to straighten the elbow. C6 adds movement of the wrist upwards, though still not use of the hands. A person may be able to transfer in and out of a wheelchair. A C7 level allows independence with elbow extension aiding transfers, though finger movements that are controlled by C8 and T1 are still not normal. For a C8 tetraplegic independence might be expected.

In thoracic injuries and below, people are paraplegic. In T1 to T8 lesions, trunk muscles as well as chest wall breathing are lost, leading to difficulties in balance in a wheelchair, which are shared with all tetraplegics. In addition, the abdominal muscle are also paralyzed, leading to the tetra tummy, a lax and large abdomen that can be so dispiriting. Lesions around T8 and below have effects mainly on leg and hip muscles.

In a complete spinal cord lesion, all sensation is lost below the level, and because people do not feel, they can injure themselves without awareness. They have to be aware of skin care to prevent burns and, especially, pressure ulcers. People in wheelchairs often do this by lifting the torso a few inches from the chair to allow temporary relief for the skin over the buttocks from the weight of the body.

The control of bladder and bowel is coordinated at S2 and below, so anyone with a complete lesion above this will be incontinent. Men usually have either an indwelling urinary catheter or introduce a cather intermittently (without sensation, of course). Women usually need the former to prevent incontinence. These increase the chances of a urinary infection, and kidney and bladder stones and renal failure must be guarded against. The bowel can be trained to empty fairly regularly, or be evacuated manually.

Sexual function is coordinated at similar levels to the bladder. Men with complete tetraplegia may experience spontaneous erections, through intact spinal reflexes in the sacral cord, but may be unable to become erect in the usual ways. Those with low sacral damage may not be able to experience erections because the local spinal and nerve reflexes are damaged. For women the lack of erection may be less of a problem than the loss of sensation.

In addition, there are a number of other functions altered or lost because of spinal cord injury. Temperature regulation can be a problem in tetraplegics, because they cannot shiver, sweat, or control blood vessels' dilatation and constriction below their level. The latter may also be the reason for autonomic dysreflexia. In these, seen in those with levels around T6 and above, large increases in blood pressure can suddenly occur, which present as severe headache and sweating over the forehead caused by dilation of the normally controlled blood vessels of the head and neck, connected to the brain by the intact cervical cord, in response to a rise in blood pressure following, say, a problem in the area of body below the level. Bladder dilation is a potent cause of this, but some people have dysreflexia during rehabilitation when they are first raised to the vertical. This is a medical emergency, with stroke a real possibility if the blood pressure is not reduced. The rise in blood pressure is all the worse because tetraplegics normally live with lower blood pressures than able-bodied people.

Muscle spasms can be a real problem in those with levels above the lumbar cord. Initially after spinal injury there is a loss of all reflex activity, known as "spinal shock." But then, over months, reflexes become abnormally active, which can lead to huge spasms in response to relatively innocuous stimuli.

Lastly, as we will see, people with spinal cord injury have to live with a variety of pain. Roughly 60–65 percent of people have pain, and in 20–25 percent it is severe. This may reflect damage to the nerve roots at the site of the lesion, or elsewhere—after all, an injury sufficient to cause cord damage may also have caused damage in the nerves in the shoulder or elsewhere. Later it may also be the result of shoulder arthritis after years of transfer from chair to car, for example. Lastly, one of the most troubling types of pain is "phantom" pain, perceived in the area of the body below the level of cord damage in an area that cannot be felt. This may be similar to phantom limb pain, as in both cases the brain is disconnected from the area in which pain is felt.

Thus the cord damage may differ in completeness, duration, and most importantly in level. Most of those I interviewed have a complete spinal cord injury in the cervical region. The neurological impairment confronts each person with a huge loss. As we will see, however, each person's response to it varies hugely.

The Simple Questions

There are many books on the science and medicine of spinal cord injury and, excitingly, more and more papers on research. But my aim was different and complimentary, to ask the simple question of what it is like to live in a wheelchair, without sensation and movement in the body. The answer is found in the experiences of those in that position, but in fact there is no single answer, for each person has different responses to their injury.

I have chosen twelve narratives of people with similar and in some cases identical impairments, but with differing experiences. How individuals responded to their new way of living has shaped the division of the book into six main sections.

It begins with the narratives of two men, each injured over twenty years ago. Though very different characters, their accounts overlap in revealing the continuing grip of spinal cord injury. These accounts may confirm something of the worst of this impairment. It seemed important, at the start, to consider tetraplegia as a huge and continuing disruption in the normal, effortless flow of life.

After these raw narratives, there is a short commentary on some aspects of the experiences of Graham and Colin. Their spinal cord injuries reveal how our bodies normally enable us to make our way in the world with little attention to them. These two men can never forget the need to care for their bodies and so never forget their spinal cord injury. It continually imposes on their waking lives, conditioning their view of the world and their view of themselves.

In the next two narratives, David and Ian, over widely dissimilar time courses, come to terms with their injuries and begin to explore ways of living. David, a young university graduate at the time of his injury, managed to live by ignoring his tetraplegia as best he could for several years before he was forced to consider it, due to illness and erroneous advice. He came through and began to explore independence and a far richer life. Ian's story, in contrast, is not over decades but over one year, and yet he too moved to an exploration of the remaining possibilities and choices open to him, with some surprises along the way.

There follows a short commentary on these two narratives, focussing on those areas raised by David and Ian's narratives. David at one stage contemplated suicide. Able-bodied readers might not find this surprising, given his tetraplegia. But, as will be seen, this thought was a response to far more complex matters than his spinal injury. After this, the experience of severe pain, which Ian has had to cope with, after injury is considered.

After such maudlin matters, it might be a surprise that both David and Ian find enjoyment and indeed some contentment in their lives. In fact, the quality of life of most people with spinal cord injury is good. They show ways of exploring and then coming to an accommodation with spinal cord injury; this forms part of the remainder of this commentary and is implicit in the remainder of the work.

These men were all well aware of how they could not inhabit their own bodies, how they could not be "in the flesh." In the next two chapters, I talk with two women who have had different functional electrical devices implanted, one to enable the return of hand function, the other, more ambitiously, for standing. The devices offer Deborah and Julie the possibility of choice and of control of parts of their bodies that were otherwise beyond their control and action. How has this affected the way they view their bodies?

Illness and impairment never affects one person alone; it always affects family and friends. The family members, though not suffering the illness, can be underinformed and left out of the loops of care and treatment. In spinal cord injury, when the patient is often in the hospital for months learning new skills and needs, this can be both an acute and an enduring problem. When the patient is also left with severe chronic pain, it can produce intolerable pressures. The next two short chapters are the recollections of two people whose spouses were injured. Unfortunately, they have differing outcomes.

The history of successful treatment of spinal cord injury is not long. Though spinal injury is recorded on papyrus scrolls, until the beginning of the twentieth century those with such an injury usually lived a few months, often rotting in side rooms of hospitals as they died of pressure sores and infection. For Sir Ludwig Guttmann, the founder of Stoke Mandeville Hospital and the pioneer of care in this area, spinal cord injury was "the most depressing and neglected subject of all medicine":

If the spinal cord is severed or crushed . . . this immediately results in a paralysis below the level of the injury, with loss of most essential functions . . . all motor functions, appreciation of all forms of sensation, and results in loss of posture and control of bladder and bowels. Sexual function in men is abolished. Women lose sexual sensation but can have intercourse and still conceive. In injuries of the cervical cord, the respiratory function as well as the blood circulation are greatly impaired, especially in very high lesions, the involvement of the blood circulation leading also to a reduction if the tone of all tissues, especially skin and muscles. This, in turn, results in a lowering of their resistance to pressure, which is one of the most important causes of the development of pressure sores.

They did not establish a social problem in the past, as their life expectancy was very short, two to three years at the utmost was the rule.[15]

Most actually lived less, with survival at the time of the First World War being a few months for most. Only 20 percent survived three years. Little happened subsequently until Guttmann arrived in Aylesbury. He found, with rigorous attention to pressure areas, to bladder infections, and to nutrition, that paraplegics (and then tetraplegics in the subsequent years) could be salvaged and given up to twenty extra years of life. But even then, as Guttmann also realized, "Most of those who managed to survive were doomed to spend the rest of their lives as pensioners at home or in institutions for incurables, dependent on other people's assistance, and as a rule, given no incentive or encouragement to return to a useful life."[16]

Following the miraculous work began by Guttmann and then taken up throughout the (developed) world, people with spinal cord injury had their lives extended by decades. But, arguably, social issues lagged behind these wonderful advances in medicine. How were people with spinal cord injury to live in society? They needed somewhere to go, because hospitals could not cope for such long periods. Many went into institutions; at the time, they were seen as a great advance, though now, for some, these homes are seen as delaying death more than prolonging life.

Over the last forty years there has been a movement, led by those with spinal cord injury themselves, for people to move from care homes to living in their own homes, either with their family or alone. Paraplegics and tetraplegics have continued their careers, allowing financial independence. This has been possible in part through the use of personal assistants at home and work. The book's next two chapters concern the narratives of two of those active in pushing for these reforms and for a move from a medical model of neurological loss and dependence to a more social and empowering one, with huge implications for how spinal cord injury is viewed. Given the energy of Stephen Duckworth and of Michael Oliver, one occasionally has to remind oneself that both are tetraplegics.

Both are also hugely eloquent, and the next chapter discusses their views on neurological impairment. The need for work as a way of gaining independence, how best to influence others to change society's view of "disability," and how the disabled can draw attention to their problems without being defined by them are debated.

After the fireworks of Stephen and Michael, the last section is quieter, deliberately so. These two chapters tell the stories of two young men who live with tetraplegia as nuisance rather than as tragedy. Nasser and

Tony's experiences reveal lives that have been able to move beyond endurance to those who manage, almost, to transcend their impairment. The lack of drama with which they relate their lives is, arguably, the most remarkable thing.

The final chapter attempts to bring some observations together and to explore some of the implications of living without movement and sensation. It is, for instance, most important to be able to manage friends and relations, familiar with you but not with spinal injury. Independence for tetraplegics is often due to the use of personal assistants. The chapter considers this curious relationship between physically active PAs and their employers. In fact, this commentary focuses on relationships: between carer and employer, tetraplegic and others, and finally tetraplegics and their altered bodies and new lives.

Talking with those with spinal cord injury and with pain, one public, one private, one an unsought absence, the other an unwanted presence, may allow different perspectives on the same thing: our relation to our bodies. Few have attempted to answer the simple questions of what it is like to live with spinal injury, because these seemed the most difficult to ask. Though I discuss theoretical and clinical aspects of the condition, it is to these simple questions that I will return again and again.

When I first encountered tetraplegics, I was fascinated by the way they carried on their lives and the ways they endured with their impairment. I spent time with some and, as guys do, discussed sport and life in general. But as a doctor doing research with them, I could never find the words or the way to talk to them about the things that interested me. I guess I was in a hurry with the research and the papers and with the next thing.

Now I have gone to people, not with a white coat or a stethoscope, and without any promise to help or assist. I have gone to listen to their lives as they express them in their own time and in their own homes. Now, I hope, I have found the words.

A Word or Two on Names

In the United Kingdom, spinal cord injury at the level of the neck and leading to paralysis of the arms, legs, and trunk is known as tetraplegia, using the Greek for loss of use of four limbs. Paralysis at the chest or lower back level leads to paralysis of the legs and some trunk muscles, sparing the arms. This is known, again after the Greek, as paraplegia. In the United States, the more familiar term quadriplegia is used, combining the Latin for four, quad, with the Greek word for paralysis. I have kept faith with the English, partly out of desire to maintain the purity of the derivation, partly out of my preferring the sound and look on the page of the T term over the Q one, and partly, others might suspect, from childish nationalism. I suspect, as in so much, that the American usage will prevail. Paraplegia can be used as a generic term for both tetra- and paraplegia. In this book I will not use this shorthand. In fact, the people whose narratives are told are all tetraplegics except for two, so one hopes this will not be confusing.

Though numbers are not a major concern, some idea of the incidence of spinal cord injury might be of relevance. It has been suggested that there are 183,000–230,000 people in the United States with such an impairment, with 82 percent male and most, 58 percent, aged between sixteen and thirty. Young people tend to be injured on roads or in violence. There may be a second peak in old age, when falls become more common.[17]

I began by talking and writing, always, of "people with tetraplegia," and never about "tetraplegics." This form of political correctness was designed to show that each person was an individual first and foremost, with his or her neurological impairment seen secondary to himself or herself. Then I met several people who were proud to be "disabled" and viewed their identities as being intimately related to their tetraplegia. They were more than happy to be defined by their impairment and to be "tetraplegics," and even were unhappy with my liberal PC use of words. So some are happy to be "people with tetraplegia" and others prefer to be tetraplegics. I have therefore used both terms and worried less. If I have used the wrong form of words in relation to a given person, I apologize.

II | Enduring

2

We Are All New Boys

Without a Mark

He had explained over the phone that he lived in the house with a picture of a steam engine on the garage. I made my way up the street half expecting to miss it, but Graham's house, a modern detached one, could not be missed. The train was as large as the garage, and looked as though it was about to roll off the wall and across the garden. I knocked at the door; Graham answered by remote and let me in. His room was large, airy, and neat, and overlooked a flat field covered by stubble and surface water, giving it a cold, wintry look; a line of electricity pylons snaked away in the distance.

Graham sat at his large, immaculate desk. I looked up; the friend who had painted the mural had decorated the ceiling with vines and trees, giving the room a slightly medieval appearance, like the Pope's chamber at Avignon.

Graham explained that he was sorry, he had not really thought too much about things for a while, and then he started.

He was twenty-two and studying quantity surveying as an external Reading University student in London. At weekends he would go home to see his parents, to have his washing done, and, of course, to party. Quantity surveying was not, after all, at the forefront of 1960s social change, and his course was almost exclusively male. At a party in Maidenhead, he had a disagreement with the girl who was driving him home. Graham was sober and thought she had drunk too much. He was not covered by her insurance, and so with misgivings, he let her drive. Three hundred yards later, at the first junction, she hit a lamppost. Graham came to in the hospital, propped up in bed.

As soon as he had recovered from the concussion, he was told he was free to go, but he found he could not move.

"A nurse said I had had concussion and could go. I woke up without a mark. It felt odd, and I realized I could only move my head. I wasn't panic-stricken; they lay me down and then started taking X-rays. After a while, the doctor came up and told me that for the rest of my life I would be a cabbage. He actually used that phraseology. I went to pieces of the spot. It was inaccurate and unnecessary."

Over the next few days in the intensive care unit, he held on as best he could. Routine became important: staff changing, meals, the cleaner coming around, all defined the day and kept Graham in touch with the world. One nurse kept telling him about her marriage breakup.

He was transferred to Stoke Mandeville Hospital near Aylesbury, the leading hospital for the care and rehabilitation of those with spinal cord injury. As soon as he arrived, callipers were inserted into his skull and he was placed flat in bed on traction. Every so often the weights on his head and neck were increased, in the hope that the neck bones would stabilize and the spinal cord recover. In fact, he only recovered a little.

Graham was given a diagnosis of complete spinal cord injury at C6/C7. He could move one triceps, flex one wrist, and bend the wrists upward. Sensation was down one side of the arms only. Walking was over.

Being in a hospital with others in the same position made life easier. He was in an old Nightingale single-sex ward, with long lines of beds in one large room. Privacy was nonexistent, but at least everyone was thrown in with each other. If anyone became depressed, they would collectively jolly him out of it, as best they could from the isolation of their beds. Those further along offered advice and care.

Graham's time at Stoke was not entirely straightforward. He was six feet tall and only weighed a hundred pounds. Being thin was a disadvantage, and he soon developed pressure sores on his sacrum, as well as various splits in the skin, despite the best attentions of the nurses. Things were not helped by some of the orderlies. Though most of the nurses were kind, they could not do all the care. In the days before hoists and lifting courses, much of the turning and washing had to be done by male orderlies, who were not always the most sensitive of individuals. Graham dreaded baths, because there was a good chance of a new split in his skin. He also developed troublesome urinary tract infections. But there was little he could do; he soon learned the balance between being compliant and popular, and the need to look after himself.

These two problems, the skin and the bladder, meant that Graham was in the hospital longer than usual, for around thirteen months. He described everything, admittedly from thirty years away, with detachment.

"I remember not being happy. I realized I would not walk and I was not going to get my hands back either, so I worked very hard to maximize what I could do. I needed to get out, go to university, and get a job. With attractive nurses and physiotherapists around, it was not that unpleasant. I had very low blood pressure and had to be sat up very, very slowly. In the early days it would take two hours at time to sit me up without passing out. Once up, your whole day was kept busy. No time to sit around and chat. I think Guttmann was right, 'Keep them busy.'[1] That element was spot on. Less time to think, and it was also fun. None of it seemed pointless."

One man at Stoke Mandeville in the early days after the Second World War, a former boxer, moaned infamously that "There's no bloody time to be ill in this bloody place."[2]

Once the skin had healed it was time for Graham to try a chair. "Because you had no sensation, it was like sitting in a wheelchair and floating. You did not feel safe in the chair in the least. This was extraordinary. Initially you could sit *in* it, but it felt like you were just a head, and so felt unstable and convinced you were going to fall out. Occasionally I did fall out, of course.

"It took weeks and months to feel OK. Now I can almost kid myself that I can feel something when I sit in a chair, even though I know I cannot. It feels exactly the same sitting in a chair now to before I was injured. It can't, but it does. My mind tells me so. My mind makes me think I am like you over there. It learns what is the norm for this body. It tells me there is nothing wrong, so I feel comfortable and correct."

For Graham, despite all the downsides, the hospital worked well and he enjoyed his time there. If you could find a nurse to take you out, they would. After the single-sex school and college, he had a good social life. There was drinking, sometimes too much, and even, for the first time in a long time, there was fun.

"My pleasure came from achieving more and the working together, like a team sport. We would bind our wheelchairs together and rush down corridors. There was a long corridor that was quite steep. We used to have to get up the hill, which was a good way of assessing strength, and in the end they put a bag of weights on me to slow me down. I was as fit as I have ever been. But you could get tired because they put on special sessions and we worked so hard. The injury, for a long time, causes tiredness in itself.[3]

"It was so positive, everything aiming for the same thing, and I was getting stronger. I was working hard without knowing what the future would hold. It was a community rather than a hospital."

Looking back, that time, for Graham, was perhaps the best he has had. The shock was coming out of hospital.

A Room of His Own

University days are portrayed as being a wonderful time when, free from parental control, you work hard—one hopes—but also play hard. Graham's college in London was 95 percent male, with no dormitories. The cheap apartments were lonely and cold. His hobby, campanology, certainly occupied some of his spare time, but ringing bells in draughty churches was hardly wild. This explains why he had been so desperate to return home at weekends for parties. His time in Stoke became better and better as he settled in, but he knew that the real world would have to be rejoined all too soon, something he awaited with a mixture of anxiety and impatience.

He was fortunate that his university department had moved to Reading and had a dorm and a health center in which he could live. He was able to return to his course, something that would have been impossible only a few years before. Once the arrangements were made, however, the problems became apparent. For one thing, he had to stay at home during vacations, even though the last thing he wanted, at twenty-two, was to be looked after by his mother.

"I did not want her near me. I was not a child. They could never understand that. They found a carer, with my father putting me to bed. It was easier with total strangers."

At the health center, he only had the strangers, with their own problems.

"It was hell. The only way they could organize it was to stay in the health center, a little room all on my own. They got me up at 6 a.m. and then back to bed at 6:30 p.m. Otherwise there would be no people to move me. It was absolutely dreadful."

It is difficult to imagine being put in bed for twelve hours a night, tired or not, unable to move. Once he went out, returned late, and was put to bed by his friends. The nurse reported him to the doctor. The doctor, fortunately, told the nurse not to be so unreasonable.

He developed a bedsore while staying with his parents during the holidays, which led to eight weeks lying flat in bed while it healed. Stuck in the health center, dependent on rotas of nurses, he questioned whether returning to university had been worthwhile. But, once healed, things looked up. He arranged a transfer to a dormitory and got to know people. The nurses remained difficult, however; one female even refused to change his urinary condom.

He persevered, ending up doing the third year twice before he got his degree in quantity surveying. He found work as a surveyor for the local County Council, passed his final exams, and became a Chartered Quantity Surveyor. He worked there for twenty-four years before reorganization, rationalization, and theoretical cost cutting made him redundant.

"Most of the time since my injury I had a full-time job. Losing my job, I don't like at all. It is partly the money, but more, perhaps, because being at home most days I feel I am in a posh prison. The loss of the job itself has not worried me, even with its loss of esteem. It's the money and the camaraderie that hit me hard. But I keep myself busy with the Parish Council. It is one the wealthiest in the country, with a budget of £100,000 per year and only 850 dwellings in the Parish. We have liquid assets of about £1.5 million. Most Parish Councils are just pressure groups, but we own two recreation grounds and two halls which we run."[4]

A Child Again

I asked about Robert Murphy's observation that, when first tetraplegic, he had had a desire to move. This seemed more than a desire for movement—it seemed that he and his movement brain wanted to command movement.

"Yes, I can certainly follow that. He is right. For me there was a frustration. You could not get up to get a glass of water. That sense of frustration has never gone. There is a permanent annoyance that you have to depend on someone else for the rest of one's life for everything. All of a sudden you are a child again."

It seemed that it was the movement actions and independence that Graham missed, rather than a more abstract feeling of wanting to move. Murphy's experience might not be exemplary; he had also made his observation soon after his illness. Graham continued, "Remember, I have been longer disabled than abled. In a relatively short time, things become a norm. You almost forget how it was before. I cannot say my brain is itching to make my legs move."

Maybe thirty years of spinal cord injury had dulled his desire to move. But other desires continued. Sexual desire, he explained, had neither disappeared nor found an outlet. Without sensation, he knew it was not going to be much fun, but a sad thing was that he had always preferred the company of women. Going to an all male school, he had never developed confidence with women; the hospital had been good for that, and then—nothing.

"I've been forced to get used to it. It does not mean that I don't miss it; I think about it and ogle every attractive woman who's around. But there is absolutely nothing I can do about it. I have not found anything. The mental imagining remains important, because I cannot feel anything. I don't get an orgasm anyway."

Some people, I said, report that they can find satisfaction from being stroked over their remaining sensate areas and may even have an orgasm.

"Good luck to them. Part of it is not sex itself, but feeling that you are a man. That's a major part of it."

The Sensation of Nothing

I was fascinated to know what it was like to live without sensation or movement. What might such an absence feel like? The obvious and frequently used analogy is having a tooth filled under local anaesthetic. One feels a numbness, with the lip feeling larger. More extraordinary is to touch the face with one's fingers; one usually feels not the fingers doing the feeling, but the touched part of the face. To touch the numb face and feel nothing is perhaps even more shocking than the numbness itself. For Graham such an analogy was unsatisfying.

"This is not the same sort of sensation somehow. . . . That numbness is sort of a void, as though something has been taken away and is no longer there. My loss of sensation is not quite like that; it is a different feeling . . ."

I said that one girl I knew had had a nerve injury with severe intermittent neuralgic pain that was so bad that it prevented her from doing anything. And yet for her, this pain—though excruciating—was not as bad as the feeling of numbness. The continual absence was worse than the pain. Wittgenstein had asked if the absence of a feeling was a feeling.[5] I asked Graham if he was aware of numbness, or of the presence of an absence? Not surprisingly, he looked back at me with some confusion.

"I have phantoms, not pain, but slight pins and needles in the feet. They feel there, though I don't know really where they are. They make me, allow me, to feel that I have a body still. The absence of sensation and feel does not feel wrong. It seems perfectly normal. Early on there was this sensation of feeling nothing and one felt disembodied, even though you knew you weren't because you could see. But you did feel completely disembodied. That was an odd sensation.

"I felt like a balloon being wafted around. It is a sensation of nothing. I immediately compared with before. To me it was a sensation. You're saying that if you can't feel you can't have a sensation. But it wasn't numbness. It was nothingness. It was a sensation because you can sense nothing. It was a definite sensation. My head floating. . . . I've never been up in a balloon, but that's how I imagine it would be."

Here Graham was comparing his entire sensation, and the effect of having a normally sentient head and neck atop a body he could not feel, with nothingness. Rather than the feeling of being in a balloon, floating in zero gravity came to mind, and the relaxation that comes from this.[6] I was fortunate a few years ago to ride on NASA's KC135 zero gravity plane, the "Vomit Comet," and found zero g a wonderful experience— so restful was it, that one did have a feeling of enjoyment and even temporary and slight euphoria (given the fact that the zero g period was only for twenty-five seconds and was followed by fifty seconds of 1.8 g).

But then I knew what was happening and could enjoy the relaxation. For Graham it was not twenty-five seconds on a plane over the Gulf of Mexico, it was permanent. I explained to Graham my time floating in the Vomit Comet.

"But that would be pleasant. This was not, it was odd and unnerving and unsafe. It's almost too long ago. Thirty years and it passed fairly quickly, because the brain now says it is a norm."

In the Vomit Comet, standing up in zero gravity, I felt an awfully long way above my body as I looked down. I wondered what it was like looking down on his body.

"It was, and is, odd, because I cannot feel it, but it still feels or looks like your own body. But then, you see, when you are just sitting down, the only sensation you have is of where you are sitting. You may be looking at your knees, but you don't actually feel them. There is no sensation as such. It did not feel so much like your body because it was not going to do what you told it to. To some extent it is an appendage, and to some extent still the same."

Graham had adapted in thirty years, and much of what he now felt was normal for him. I changed the subject a little. I liked running, for the physical release and oneness I felt with my body. Did he have any understanding of this immersion in movement?

"Two years ago, I bought a tracker [a tricycle moved with arm cranks], and I must admit that I have had more pleasure out of it than from any thing else since I have been disabled. I am cycling, going from one place to another under my own control. I am amazed at how much pleasure it is giving me. I did it simply to get a bit of exercise. I disappear off on my own, and because I am working and exercising. It almost feels as though I am not disabled."

By controlling and enjoying his own body and, through that, by moving though the world, he was connected with his body in a manner he had not been for years.

The Screaming Tree

I asked about anger—not about his feelings about the injury, but how he expressed it. Anger, after all, is a body thing as much as anything. Merleau-Ponty had even written that "the gesture does not make me think of anger, it is anger itself."[7] Was the quality of anger the same before as after?

"Becoming disabled adds another element to be angry about. Anger does not involve, or require, throwing something across the room. It is in the mind, and I don't think anger needs external expression. I have always tended to express it internally; otherwise, it is counterproductive. I read a wonderful book which had a screaming tree in it. Each time you are angry, you could go out and scream at it. Wonderful. Anger, though, is the same.

"I don't do it very often because it is counterproductive. But with one professional carer, I did shout at her. She was not doing her job. I still wave my arms around. Sometimes I feel it more, since anger can be borne of frustration, and therefore it can multiply. The first carer who looked after me must have suffered hugely. That anger was out of frustration, not bitterness. Any sense of religious belief disappeared with my injury.

"I feel for those who are less academic. I was a pen pusher and always was going to be. But manual workers just have to sit at home. Many marriages break up, usually because the disabled person pushed their spouses away, saying they were unworthy. Whether they wanted to or not, they did it deliberately.

"Your whole mental approach differs completely. You are not the same person. You think differently. . . . You are a young man, twenty-two or twenty-three, with your whole life ahead of you, hoping for a wonderful time, then a career. All things are possible, all things are there. Then, all of a sudden, circumstances dramatically change and there is absolutely nothing you can do about it except tinker around the edges, however you may rail against it. That has a terrible effect. You start thinking what is the point of it all if you cannot run your own life.

"Once you have recognized this fact, then you cannot be the same person because you don't have the same hope. You cannot say I am going to do this, because you have no chance of doing it. Your attitude alters; this cannot be hidden.

"It also changes the way you see the world and the way you see others. You don't see in the same way. The world is not your oyster, it is actually crushing in on top of you. It is pushing you in and you cannot get out. Life becomes claustrophobic. Endless things you can't do—all of a sudden you are confined to what others will let you do, what society will allow you to do.[8]

"I wanted to get out because I had less opportunity and less chances to. I can never have enough friends or see them enough. I never, and have never, felt less of a person than before. In that sense I am the same as I was before, except for the way it has changed me. . . . Without control you are a totally different person. You view the world differently and the world views you differently. People know me as being in a wheelchair, *as* a wheelchair. I always try to put myself on the other side. If I were looking at me, I am sure I would be thinking of that guy in the chair. I can't expect them to think any differently.

"I must admit I can't really claim that I have ever been happy or content since I have been in a wheelchair. The frustrations have always been there to take it away. For me each day, life is either bearable or unbearable. It has never really got beyond that. Very few days have got above bearable.

"Happiness is a positive emotion, short-term enjoying a film, an overall feeling. Before I was disabled I was sometimes happy and sometimes not, but since I have been disabled I cannot claim that I have ever been happy. It is too much of a struggle, every day."

I wondered if he could distract himself from the realization, the presence of his tetraplegia. Might reading transport him somewhere else? If not that, then films, television, anything?

"I can be immersed in reading, but it is too short term for me to say that this makes me happy. A good book will take me to places that even a film might not. You are right. I tend to have batches of book reading. Before I was disabled, I was an avid reader, but since then I have less time. I do enjoy it. . . . But I cannot leave my disability completely. It is too short a time.

"I guess you could take drink or drugs to escape reality. But I cannot. So it is always there, when I shut the book, or put the top back on the bottle, reality is there. It never leaves, except when asleep. Some dreams I remember, and though a number are unpleasant, I am usually not disabled. What, I wonder, of the dreams of those born disabled?"

A Landslip

"My hobbies before were vintage cars and sailing. Both physical. I miss them still. A pain is that there is so much I would like to do but can't, and it is getting worse, not better, because of the Health and Safety Acts. I used to go on steam rail tours, but they won't take me now. On boats they previously offered to put me in a bag and crane me across. This is no longer permitted; things that interest me are being closed. At work I had a terrible time because, after many years of people helping me transfer from my car, they suddenly announced that there was no one to lift me out of the car, in case someone was injured and could sue the Council. In the end the Council sent people on 'lifting' courses so that they could get me out of my car—something they had already been doing for many years.

"Now I have more time but less I can do. Things I may have done when first in a chair, they will not let me do. You are being told things are getting easier for us, but they are not. The care element is difficult. Carers are not around; they are looking after younger people or even the older people."

I came back to the changes in perception of his body and of his sense of self after the injury, and more especially now, after three decades. From talking with Graham it was clear that much of what he experienced was normal—normal for him. In this sense, he was not disabled but able—and sentient—in different ways.

"I just feel me. Me is the mental side. I am what I think, rather than I am what I do. I release my thoughts into speech or writing or anything else, rather than into any other movement. It is still doing, but less doing. It is more intellectual, but that is one reason why I enjoy that cycling, because it is a raw physical release. Before I did not realize how badly I needed it.

"But I do accept that my mind has changed. My total viewpoint and mental processes are different, and these cause a major change in personality. Everyone changes as they grow, age, and experience life. But this is more like a landslip; everything changes in one go.

"I can say why, but not easily how. I feel I have changed because of the physical limitations, because everything has to be planned much more carefully, and because of a hundred and one other things. I think in a totally different way. I have to plan every day, with little spontaneity. I cannot just decide to go out. It has to be calculated, and this affects the way I think and my character. But how to define this? Character is what you are. How you behave, how you act, how you think, how you cooperate with others.

"How you act is physical, I accept, but character is mental. But the physical has a knock effect on everything. Everyone changes and evolves, but here it happens in one big jolt. Sixty years ago we would have all died. We are all new boys.[9] It is amazing that we cope quite happily."

I suggested they cope by keeping busy, as Guttmann had suggested.

"He was spot on. If you spend too long thinking, you'll get fed up. But that is similar for anyone, able bodied or not. I can't help feeling that many people with tetraplegia die off early out of boredom and frustration and because they are not achieving anything. Because of this, they don't care for themselves sufficiently well. Of those I was in the hospital with, there is only one whom I know is still alive. And that one I do know is in a bad state. My life expectancy was twenty-five years, so I have exceeded it by five years so far."

A Nightmare of Carers

Those with spinal cord injury now have a choice about where they live. Until recently, they lived either at home with family carers or a "home," purpose built to care for "the disabled."[10] These were run with the best of intentions, and gave many people opportunities they would not otherwise have had. But for most with spinal injury, the regimented care was less than ideal. A third possibility, increasingly, is to live independently with a team of carers or personal assistants to help with dressing, feeding, washing, and so on. Some years ago, when Graham was considering this, however, there were some snags. His consultant in Stoke once asked him whether he was homosexual or heterosexual.

"Heterosexual, thank you, sir."

"That's bad luck: You'll have a much better time if you are homosexual. I advise you never to employ a male carer, because a lot of those that do the caring are either alcoholics or homosexuals, and you won't know until it's too late."

Because he preferred being looked after by women, that was fine. Graham has, over thirty years, had a succession of carers, some good, some bad. It is the less successful he remembers.

"My life has been made worse by them. Some have been real nightmares. This is a consequence of being disabled, but magnified as a consequence of being in a wheelchair. You never know how long they will last, and then they are not cheap. This has been by far the most difficult element. My life has completely turned around such that life is survival rather than anything else."

I mentioned that, as a disabled person, one is not allowed to be glum. Robert Murphy has written, "A key rule for being a successful sick person is don't complain."[11]

"That is spot on. It is rather the other way around. You don't gain anything from being down. It is noticeable that if I do get depressed, my carers have all wanted to leave. I go very quiet and don't want to say anything."

I thought that carers might have thought that part of their role might be to cheer him up, rather than taking their mood from Graham.

"It does not seem to work like that. Whenever I get fed up, they get really fed up too. Most of the time I am a relatively happy soul. If I was not, then life would be much more difficult. One carer used to put me to bed and then would talk to me for two hours. She just would not go, and this drove me to distraction. I tried to ask her to leave the room, but she would not. That is one of the problems; your carers have full control. You cannot do a damn thing about it. That's when frustration and anger kick in. Eventually she took notice of my screams and she would go."

But he also realized the difficulties for the carers. "It's not easy for a carer. I am the only one here, and it can be very constraining for them."

As his consultant had intimated, the work may attract certain people. I wondered how he ever terminated their employment.

"It can be very difficult. One went to London one night and was not back till 10 a.m. the next day. I was due at work at 9 a.m. I tried to throw her out, and she said she'd nowhere to go and holed herself up in her room. It took me a month to get her out. The police were not interested, said it was domestic. I had invited her in the first place. I couldn't get her out, though eventually she went.

"You also get weirdoes. One woman may have been a man. Just as well, he was the ugliest woman I have ever seen, and a complete liar as it turns out. He left to look after children, and the mother phoned me up later to ask if I knew him/her and said she thought he'd been molesting the kids. I even had the police around. He left behind this huge number of birth control pills, which I understand can be used for hormone replacement. Someone else forged checks.

"When you are on your own, you are on your own.

"It's a minority like that, but a significant one. You cannot rely on agencies. I'll stick with them while I have the money. But the cost is around £25,000 per year, and I cannot survive that long on that. So I don't know how some people needing carers manage, especially if they are not married. It's always in the back of your mind that there will be a time when I cannot afford a carer and then . . .?"

By now we had talked out. His Filipina carer had come back, and it was time for attending to other things. I made to go. He relaxed and, as he did, he came back to sex, saying that—even now—sexuality and sex was for him a huge matter.

"For someone who is disabled, to have a partner is almost more important than for an able-bodied person. God, it is important enough anyway. I have been unlucky on that score, and that has made everything that much more difficult. I've never had anybody as a soul mate, and that is the difference between being content and being not content."

When I was with Graham, I listened to an almost academic account of life with tetraplegia; once on the page, I saw the enduring rawness of his feelings after nearly thirty years of spinal cord injury. I had no idea whether or not he was typical, so I went to see Colin, who was a similar age to Graham and had had a similar length of time since his injury.

3

I Do Not Live a Normal Life

Cramming Things In

It was winter, and by the time I got to Colin the light had faded. I knocked on the door and his mother started to answer, only for Colin to take over. He showed me to his room, with his bed in one corner and his desk and television next to it. He was in his late forties, and a big man. Introductions were short, and before he started talking, he lifted his legs onto the bed to prevent swelling. He adjusted them continually as he talked.

His childhood was an active one. Despite him being academic, it was clear that he had preferred doing to thinking.

"I crammed a huge amount of things before the accident. We never had money. I was born after the war and can remember rationing, so I wanted some money. From age twelve, I had a paper route, by thirteen, I had a morning one and an evening one and two Sunday ones. I had a motorized scooter before I was sixteen, and renovated it myself; I wanted mobility. By fourteen, every holiday, summer, Christmas, and Easter, I worked in a timber yard, as a fitter's mate maintaining woodworking machinery, saws, planers, pole dressing machines, steam cranes, and a tarmacadam plant—all this before I was sixteen."

He was very athletic and enjoyed football and cricket at his primary school. He passed the entrance examination for the local grammar school. By thirteen, he was playing rugby and cricket for the school team, then playing football for a local club on Sunday, and horse riding. With schoolwork as well there was little spare time, though he always found time for girls.

At the yard he sometimes worked behind the desk, dealing with people who were none too savory. Later, he remembers foreign boats delivering timber to the docks. The sailors would arrive, unload, and get drunk. Once he was asked to help quell some trouble by an old night watchman. It is not surprising that he found school comparatively dull. But he knew he had to stick at it and, despite all his other work, did not find it difficult. He was expected to apply for university, but wanted to get on with his life and so opted for day release training with an electronics firm. He did not need a degree to do what he wanted: making things, doing things.

Then everything changed forever.

He was nineteen, and had been working and playing hard, burning the candle at both ends. He worked shifts and, in his spare time, managed rugby, or cricket in the summer, swimming and playing golf. He also loved horse riding and that day had spent the afternoon at a pony race. In the evening he was driving his girlfriend home when an argument developed about another girl he had been talking to at the race. He overtook a car, heated up from the argument; as he overtook, the steering seemed to go and, possibly because of a crosswind, the car turned over. The top of the car disappeared, and Colin found himself on the grass verge.

"I remember laying there, spitting glass out, aware that people were asking if I could feel. I could not move and was incapable of feeling anything. I don't know if I was groggy or not. Then an ambulance and someone saying, 'You'll be alright' as they do."

He was taken to the local hospital. His father arrived and looked at Colin, "as though I was dead." At one stage they did not think he would survive the night. He spent two weeks in intensive care, oblivious to what was going on. When he began to come around from the injury and the sedatives, he had a calliper in his head pulling the neck; he had fractured the cervical spinal column at C6/C7. He was transferred to a Stryker frame, which allowed him to be turned "like meat on a spit," and so prevented pressure sores. This was the most terrifying thing. Incapable of moving, he was either on his back or on his front, able to look only at the floor or the ceiling for seven weeks. He could neither feel nor move below the neck.

On several occasions he was angry when, at visiting time, they would not turn him onto his back so that he could see his family. Half the time he watched the floor. He was told that they had put the neck back and there was a good chance he would have a full recovery. Then, after ten weeks, his consultant came around and told him the damage was permanent. In the end, a little recovery occurred within the first few months; some arm and hand movement returned, with scrambled sensation that changed from day to day, but nothing else.

Graham had spoken about his life with a rather detached air, as though it had happened long ago and almost to someone else. Colin, in contrast, was living it again as he spoke, hardly looking at me and pausing only to move his legs.

"You can't imagine how devastating this was when you've just turned twenty. And that they can't do anything about it. Absolutely nothing. You cannot imagine the anger, the grief, and the devastation I was living with."

He spent three months in the local hospital, gaining a reputation as a rebel, unable to deal with the discipline, desperate to come to terms with his injury. There was no one with experience of patients with spinal cord injury, no psychological care or support. More prosaically, it was not until he was transferred to Stoke Mandeville that he was treated for a bladder infection.

He could not even sleep. Dependent now on his diaphragm for breathing, lying on his stomach was a terrifying experience, struggling for breath. After seven weeks of lying down, they tried him in a wheelchair. He immediately fainted, and it was a further two weeks before he managed to sit.

Stoke Mandeville suggested a way out, and he clung to that hope of better care and some recovery, but the transfer there was very uncomfortable. Lying on a stretcher in the back of an ambulance, not knowing which way it would move next as it went around corners, he rolled backward and forward without control. The journey was a slow nightmare.

Once there he did not feel welcome. They liked to take people from the start, and he was a late arrival. Still angry and frustrated, he did not endear himself to them. The orderlies were North African and treated him quite rudely; when he protested, they threatened to send him back.

He did settle in, though, and found some good things. He liked the intensive and regimented physiotherapy. Each day was set out on a 9 to 5 basis, like school, with each hour allocated. They played as well as worked, with sports such as table tennis and basketball encouraged—these taught hand and arm use better than just doing exercises. Guttmann's idea of occupying patients the whole time, not giving them time to think, worked for Colin. The days flew by.

Despite this, he could not wait to get out. He found the atmosphere and the constant reminder of his new condition and new nature oppressive. It stopped him from doing anything and, more than that, smothered his very soul.

"I could not do anything. It is a shocking situation to deal with. I deal with it, even now thirty years later, but I cannot come to terms with it. I never come to terms. I just had too much of a life, too much to live for that no amount of counselling or patronizing could help. I got so angry, I wanted to do so much more. I could not screw a woman. I couldn't repair the car, I could not even wash it."

A perfectionist, for him to see others doing things he was once capable of doing better himself only intensified the frustration and anger. My thoughts turned to the sport he so enjoyed.

"You just cannot substitute for the experience of being able to use this wonderful piece of equipment, the body, be it running, riding, or shagging. My greatest passion was horse riding. The sheer enjoyment and freedom of being able to go hell for leather across the forest on the back of this living being with communication and some measure of control, but not too much. It was awe-inspiring and wonderful and something that I cannot ever experience again. People say why not go to 'Riding for the Disabled.' I don't want to sit on a horse and be led round a fucking paddock. That's nothing compared to what I was doing.

"I enjoyed contact with a whole body experience, like rugby. It is the sheer total involvement and the physical contact. I play basketball or table tennis, but it is not the same, not an experience which is satisfying because it is done on a restrictive basis, and you cannot throw yourself into it.

"I can never forget that I am in a chair. I am devastated by my body now. It was wonderful. . . . I used to go to rugby circuit training—twenty minutes of intense effort. I used to crawl out of the gym on my hands and knees and puke. But then I felt great that I could do these things. Now I get none of this."

I mentioned Robert Murphy's experience of how, soon after his becoming tetraplegic, he had an intense desire to move but how, with time, the will to move decayed, leaving him with a continued intellectual sense of loss, but with, at least, some peace.

"No. Not for me. Every time I am in bed I try to move something. Every time. I desperately try to move something. I have to try to deal with it, but I just cannot accept my situation, I cannot. I know it's real, but I don't want to live with it, to be honest.

"I have to accept and to live in the real world; you cannot delude yourself forever. But I try to have some hope, and always there is an expectation that it might change. I am realistic enough to know that, if by some miracle, the lesion in my neck were to heal I would be faced with so many other problems in degeneration of the body that it would be a nightmare. It is always a hope that something, however small, might improve. And that keeps you going. It must. The option is . . . you can't give up and die, for society will not let you; they will try to save you, whatever state you are in. Euthanasia is not an option in this country.

"I would have done it years ago. There is absolutely no doubt in my mind. If I could lay my hands on a guaranteed instant solution to death, I would take it. This is a living nightmare, and the reason one doesn't is that there is always the danger that you would not succeed. I do not want to do this as a cry for help. I want to do it and make sure it works. If I were to lay my hands on a handgun now, for example, like I could if I lived in the States, then after a few pints of beer, I would be gone. I would know it would be the end. I am always terrified that the job would not get finished, and I do not want that to happen.

"I think it would have been a lot kinder on my family if I had died at the time of my accident. I have tried desperately over the years to try to become reconciled, to make it rational and accept and go forward with what I have left, but I cannot."

There was a long silence; Colin was alone somewhere in his own private hell. He was not opening out for me, but to me. I had asked him before if he really wanted to talk and offered to talk about something—anything—else. He had refused; it was important to tell his story. I respected him, but had not anticipated such rawness. Colin, after all, had lived for thirty years with his injury, he had a job and was living fairly independently with his parents. By most measures he had done well.

I was unsure whether to try to say something comforting or try to change the mood. But I did not think Colin wanted the latter; he was trying to tell it like it was for him, not as he might have to talk to friends or family, or even to his doctors. His anguish was as painful and tormented as I imagined it had been when he was first injured.

Knowing that for many people with spinal cord injury movement becomes of lesser importance, I asked quite why it was so important for him.

"I am amazed you say that. Can you not imagine how dependent you are on other people? It is so devastating. And that's just talking about movement. What about all the other things? The double incontinence, the impotence. You lose so much."

I explained that my remark was not so facile. I tried to make Colin see how for others in his position movement itself was not necessarily a huge thing, though I accepted that the other problems were.

"The lack of movement dominates my life totally. Nothing is effortless. I want to—I am happy to—describe and to make it explicit. I see films about disability and think, 'Come on, you are not telling us the real stuff. How does he do his bloody bowels and how does he pee?' But there's no point doing that. People would walk out, no one would watch."

It was late, and I was exhausted by the intensity of his narrative. He was tired too, as well he might be. I sat and slowly talked of nothing, of football and of cricket, things we could share. He seemed available for this, and after a while it was time to go.

When next I saw Colin he had just recovered from a serious bladder infection. Though spinal cord injury is one of the most disastrous single insults one could imagine, it is not really a single medical event. Most people need repeated medical assessment and follow up, and frequent interventions. He had just had an abscess removed from between the legs. They had also found an obstruction in the urethra and asked him to come back for a cystoscopy and a bladder neck incision. He refused. This reluctance was not partial or negotiable. He was terrified of further surgery. Every time he had had an intrusive procedure over the last few years, he had ended up with another infection. But there was another reason for his reluctance.

He just could not come to terms with going back in. This filled him with dread, even for checkups. He had managed to stay out for nearly thirty years. To have to go back to the hospital meant going back to when he was first injured, seeing those in for the first time. To be on a ward and to be an in-patient was torture. He was, he explained, literally terrified at the prospect.

"It is not just the risk of infection. It is the whole thing. The culture. . . ."

Going back terrified him, but he was also fearful of the here and now. Once in the hospital, despite the care of nurses and physiotherapists, he lost what little precious control he had over daily living.

"I don't think people understand that once my wheelchair is taken away I am effectively shackled and chained. I have no power to do anything. The most disabling things for me in hospital are the nurses, and the way in which they attend to me. They do not understand. I organize and plan every movement I make in some detail. Not only to prevent too much effort, but also to make sure I do not have to rely on others. If I put things in a particular order in a locker, I put them there for a reason. Then a nurse comes along and quite unthinkingly moves the locker and does not put it back. Then I have to demand more of her time, or someone else's time, to move it all back again. Every time I move around, I just do not think I have got to go there. I think what else can I do either on the way or on the way back, which will save me making another trip.

"I evacuate my bowels in the evening. In the hospital I was assured my normal routine would be adhered to, but then, after trying to do it this for a couple of days, I had to give up. There were not enough staff. Everyone else had it done in the morning, and so I had to fall in with that. I conceded defeat.

"I would like to be constructive. It is trying to get across to them that though they work in a specialist unit, they are not the experts, I am."

Those who live with chronic neurological problems should be experts in their own condition but, equally well, it may be hard for nurses to be able to juggle the competing demands of many patients simultaneously.

Listening to Pain

We had reached a break, and Colin's mother appeared with some tea. We drank and relaxed a little. I asked about what remaining sensation he had.

He explained that this was bizarre. Because it had been static for so long he was used to it, and had worked out what the various signals meant. The easiest one was when he needed a bowel movement. This produced a sensation somewhere in the abdomen best described as a fullness. Occasionally he could, he thought, feel the sphincter contracting, too. But this did not mean he had control, just that he had a warning. Sometimes the feeling came but nothing came of it—a cruel phantom. He also knew when his legs were cold by an ache deep in his bones and some hot/cold differentiation, but again this was a feeling rather than a clear sensation. He could feel some pressure and tightness; pressure on his backside where a lot of the pain came from.

He lived with different sensations buzzing around that had little relation with what was actually going on. Normal for Colin was when he could feel nothing.

If there was nothing, I wondered, was that numbness?

"Numbness is, I suspect, exactly what a normal person feels, receiving messages and sensations like trousers touching the leg, when the brain adapts and filters them out. Something you don't want to be attending to all the time. My sense of numbness is not all the time or all places. Over the thigh is nearly completely numb, but there is always something. If numb, you would not be aware, say, that the feet are there. I am always aware that they are there, due to abnormal sensations."

I felt some relief that he was able to discuss these aspects more dispassionately. I asked if these sensations were painful.

"Pain is quite a subjective thing. Some experiences you might consider painful at one time and less so at another. It just becomes discomfort because you are so used to it and you cope with it. I have pain constantly. Barely a day goes by without pain."

As with many other people with spinal cord injury, I had had to ask directly about pain before it was volunteered. Colin lived with pain but rarely talked of it.

"Anyone suffering pain for any length of time will get fed up. Will this ever stop? Will I have it for the rest of my life? Will I ever be able to cope with it? Is there any way of relief? It is everywhere. It changes daily: ankles, buttocks, feet, internally in the gut, almost every day around the shoulders due to the stress of transfers. I have had six cortisone injections and have taken anti-arthritis medication but it was not doing much good and was affecting my guts. Six days a week, all day, I have pain. I might be lucky one day."

I plucked a long series of adjectives to describe pain: burning, stabbing, cramping. I asked which of those fitted?

"All of those, especially burning and stabbing. Since I had had dysreflexia several times, I know what real pain is. If I put dysreflexia at ten, the worst, then the shoulders are at an eight and my backside is around seven."

It must be exhausting to have pain for long periods.

"I can bear any pain. I bore the pain of dysreflexia for three weeks. It dilates the blood vessels in the head and gives you an enormous headache. Unless it is treated with anti-blood pressure drugs, the blood vessels in the brain don't go back and so are susceptible to any subsequent increase in blood pressure. Any strain, like the bladder or the bowels, may set it off.

"If the pain becomes so bad I cannot stand it, then I tend to focus on something else, say an impossible problem at work, or an answer to a mind game, focussing on it completely. Thinking of going to relaxing places, descent techniques, do not work for me. You just get used to it. What is the option?"

I wondered if he could distract himself from the pain or even if he might be able to forget, temporarily at least, the spinal injury.

"Never. I never can get in a position where I am comfortable and in which I can relax for a couple of hours. I always have to think and be constantly aware that there is a slight pain in the buttocks and I have to protect the skin. There is always something somewhere to remind me of the condition.

"I have to be vigilant. Fortunately, because I have as much sensation as I have, I don't have to think, because my body tells me. I would rather have it that way. When I had the first cystoscopy, they gave me a spinal anesthetic which completely numbed the body from the waist down. I found that a very difficult situation. I was totally unaware, had lost all spatial awareness of my lower body, and then things like transfers were very, very difficult because I did not know where I was.

"I would probably prefer to live with the discomfort and the pain than not to have any sensation. The prospect of having a pressure sore is too bad to contemplate."

Colin considered whether, if given the choice, he would prefer numbness to the discomfort and pain. Even if his body did not need the protection that some pain provided, then he would still prefer the awareness, though it was very difficult. He would sooner put up with the pain than lose, say, some awareness of the bowels and have a mishap.

"Most of the sensation I listen into usefully is pain. I also suffer from severe spasms, and when they go off it is very painful. But I would not give up my spasms. I can prepare myself for the pain, and it's only brief, but I can cope. Alcohol reduces them. Over the years I have tried to analyze when they come. If something does not happen as before, I am always trying to think why that should have been the case and what I can do to correct it. Is it diet or behavior? I am always analyzing what I do, and how I do it, to try and reduce discomfort and pain. I do not live a normal life."

A Normal Day

"I wake up. Then it's struggling to get myself moving. After so many years, it is getting more difficult, especially if, for once, you find yourself feeling quite comfortable in bed. Eventually I stir myself and then heave myself up in bed and put on my urinal sheath, which takes some working out when the hands are not as good as they used to be. Then I can get myself dressed, heave myself into a chair, into the bathroom, taking all the bits and pieces, emptying the bottles and disinfecting them. I wash and shave, and this takes the best part of an hour.

"My parents share the house with me, so both are usually up, and breakfast is quite painless. I scan the paper as I eat and then clean the old gnashers. Coat on, out the door, to garage (remote door), into car, and transfer and drive off to work. This all takes around two hours, with the journey being thirty minutes or so. Take chair out of car and reassemble it. This is excruciating painful because of my shoulder. Then off to work, where I spend the next eight hours or so, sat at a screen usually.

"I leave work at 5:30–6:30 p.m. and drive home. Generally my meal is ready within half an hour or so, so we eat around 7 p.m. Then I have a cup of coffee, some booze, and a smoke in the conservatory. Last year I went into hospital and the young doctor asked me the usual questions, and I said I smoked. She was horrified and said that I must stop. The bottle of wine each day, often supplemented by three or four pints of beer, horrified her. Why, I replied, should I care?

"I am very disciplined and never smoke in the house. Then I watch the TV for an hour or two. Then it's the nightly ritual of attending to the bowels. This is usually an hour minimum, and can take two. With my rectal prolapse this makes it more difficult. I manually evacuate.

"Then I take off my urinary sheath and wash myself down there and sterilize the bags and bottles and bring it all into the bedroom. The hardest thing to deal with is the incontinence. The transfer pain is predictable; the incontinence is not. Because I was rehabilitated at Stoke thirty years ago, I lie on my side and then lay my penis in a bottle at night. One has to be very careful to avoid movement and cause a disaster.

"At the weekend I catch up with all the paperwork to run a house, and I read the paper a little more than I used to."

He was finished. Keen to explore other things, I asked what he enjoyed.

"What, now? Nothing. Not a lot anyway. Driving to work is the most normal thing. It is about the only thing which might be fun, if I could go as long as I wanted. I have to be aware of my bladder and bowels and sitting properly. I always fill up at the local station and pay five to six pence per liter more to go to a station with an attendant.

"I can see humor in the world, but—and I know it sounds very self-centered—but I am so angry and bitter at having the pleasures of the world taken from me at such an early age. I can watch a good film or have a few beers, but am never taken out of myself, I always have to be aware. I have heard it, and have read it, and I cannot believe it, that some people have said that their lives have been enhanced by having a spinal cord injury. I find it difficult to accept that concept."

In his bedroom were pictures of women, and I glanced at them. Colin picked up on what I was thinking.

"The desire is still there. Absolutely. And with no release. I always was, and still am, a very sexually motivated person. I can still indulge in foreplay and all sorts of touchy stuff, but have no ability to reach orgasm or ejaculate. The absence of that overwhelming sensation of pleasure and release afterwards is something I never, ever, have got over. I don't think anyone who is able bodied and has experienced orgasm can understand what it must be like not to experience it. Constant desire but not able to get any release. . . . Just as not being able to ride across the forest or crash into someone at rugby. I will never get used to it."

After his injury, he had met a girl with whom he was in love with and planned to marry. Then it dawned on him that to inflict his pain and anger on somebody he cared so much for would be grossly unjust, so he finished with her. This act, at least, offers him some comfort, and he hopes she found happiness elsewhere. But he still regrets it and feels that maybe he would have approached it differently five or ten years down the line, once he had lived with the injury more.

A Voyeur

A few weeks later, we met again. The sun was going down, and when I arrived Colin was sitting in the conservatory, finishing a cigarette and catching the last light of the day. England had just won a Test Match at cricket, against the world number one side, Australia, against the run of play on a spectacular last day. I had driven from work as the highlights were on TV and, knowing of his love of the game, asked if he had watched. He answer was no; he knew the result and could not watch recorded sport. I felt sorry that he could not find some boyish enthusiasm for such a day. We chatted and, as it grew colder, we went into his bedroom once more.

I tried to suggest that, in the absence of movement, he might develop an intellectually based self-confidence rather than one based on a lost physicality. Colin was aware of this, "but intellectual confidence can only be fulfilled and expressed in the company of people at the same intellectual level. When one's world is populated by people at a much lower intellectual level, then it becomes impossible. I may have confidence in my intellectual level, but it cannot be expressed or enjoyed except in certain elitist company. Then I am a match in confidence for anyone, but in day-to-day living one does not mix like that. There is no solace in being bright. You come across as arrogant."

I thought of Chekhov's characters trapped far from Moscow. I asked about watching others—was there any way this could transport him and allow him to participate as others do?

"I cannot get involved in the same way. If you go to a football match, you are standing up and down, waving and cheering. I cannot do that.

I feel that loss of involvement and engagement desperately. There is a huge barrier between me and other people. I cannot gain from others. I merely watch sport or an erotic movie as a voyeur. You are in some way participating, but I do not feel that."

Concerned that we had always met after work, when we were both tired, I suggested going out, maybe a football match, something that might be fun. But in the winter, the cold gave him spasms of the legs, so we settled for lunch in a pub.

I wheeled him there with some nervousness, partly because I was mindful of his problems being wheeled and partly because the pub entrance was difficult in a chair. Once there, he was more relaxed, though I did not get many marks for driving.

He had had a recent problem in the bath. On the way out, he had trapped one leg under him and slumped forward; his mother had had to help him out. He subsequently worked out that the best way was to fill the bath more so that he could float to the top and so reduce the need for a clamber/transfer out. I suggested a hoist would be easier. Colin agreed it might be useful, but did not want one. He would overcome it his way. A simple piece of machinery would enhance his quality of life hugely, but to him that would be giving in, despite his bad shoulder pain from so many transfers. We disagreed as we ate.

As we chatted, I was fascinated by his gestures, which were busy and animated.[1] But Colin's were all down by his side, in part to avoid overbalancing in the chair, I knew, but also because his shoulders were so painful.

Transfers seemed to be a real problem. To lift his dead weight on the arms several times a day had worn away his shoulder joints. In addition, each time he transferred, he had to throw himself from chair to car, or chair to bed, uncertainly and riskily. Recently he had missed his bed, last thing at night, and ended up on the floor. Fortunately his sister was staying and he was able, just, to get a phone and call her to help. Even then he, at over six feet tall and two hundred pounds, was not easy to get into bed.

We chatted on as the beer went down.

"The last holiday I had was in 1984, to Florida. Now I just have time off; the forest and me. I sit out and enjoy what sun there is, in the peace and tranquillity of the forest.

"I am as angry as before. With most conditions these days there is always some reason for hope or optimism. But in spinal cord injury it doesn't matter which specialist you ask. They answer, 'Not in your lifetime.' The only thing to look forward to is the fact that it is going to get progressively worse. To manage that is very difficult.

"Sleep is the closest to death. You are not conscious, are you? It takes an effort because of the pain and discomfort in the shoulders and hips. I have not had a complete night's sleep for thirty years. I used to set the alarm to turn over half way through, but now I always wake up. And I have to be careful to change over the bottle as well.

"I was proud of my physical stature when I was young and fit. Now I have not come to terms with my body. Can you accept that this is your lot and you have to make your new life? I cannot. I cannot come to terms with what to me is, and was, my life being taken away from me. And, much as I try to find a substitute or alternative, it is not good enough. Not being able to do the silly things you did before. Now everything is a struggle; everything is conscious."

We sat and enjoyed a drink and a meal, Colin relaxing in the warm bar in the company of his pub friends. I knew that he would have disclosed none of his private world to them. The barman helped us out of the pub and I wheeled Colin back home. As I was leaving, I said that I hoped to get as close to the experience of living with spinal cord injury as possible. It was a chilling moment when he shot back, "Try it."

4   Endurance

A Serious Student of Myself

It was not only doctors who cautioned me against asking people with spinal cord injury about their experiences. Some paramedical staff on the wards said the same. It would only make people think too hard about their condition. "We never ask. . . ." Their sentences tailed off. One physiotherapist said how hard each day had been for her, seeing the young men so affected. The silence of paramedical and medical workers was not simply to protect the patients; it was to avoid getting too close.

Many people might have expected answers and experiences similar to those of Graham and Colin. I had expected the obvious division of their lives into two by their accidents—no one forgets that day, a cruelly lit flashbulb of memory. Robert Murphy had written, "My past is divided into two parts: pre-wheelchair and post-wheelchair. I think of the pre-illness years as a golden age. . . . My history is no longer smooth or linear, but bisected and polarized."[1]

But still the power of their words had surprised me. Similar though their stories might appear, there were many differences, too. Graham's words were delivered almost apologetically and dispassionately, almost as though he was a student of his own life. In contrast, Colin's words had a rawness and passion. He regarded himself a spectator, unable to submerge himself in experiences, even though his frustration and anger, even after thirty years, were fresh and eloquent. There is, however, another way in which those with spinal cord injury are students.

Normally we run, sit, eat, talk, with little attention to the body that allows us to act in the world. It just does what we want, what we need, what we are. Our bodies seem phenomenologically absent from our attention for much of the day. Shaun Gallagher[2] and Drew Leder[3] have written about the ways in which the body is perceptually transparent for much of our daily lives. Merleau-Ponty wrote that "I observe objects, but not my own body."[4] Leder uses the example of leaning against a picket fence and gazing on a sycamore tree, unaware of standing or leaning. We have all been walking along a street, stumbled, and then become aware of our body. When things are unexpected, when there is a mismatch between what we ask the body to do and what actually happens, our attention is drawn toward it, by vision or by sensory feedback.[5] We quickly reestablish our balance and so direct attention outward again, maybe to whatever led us to stumble in the first place.

It is clear that without sensation and movement, tetraplegics are not freed from their bodies. In fact, it is almost the opposite: they have to attend constantly in a different way to their bodies, trying to interpret what little they are aware of, trying to find meaning in vague sensations. Does this sensation mean a bladder evacuation is likely, or a bowel movement? Does heel pain mean I could be at risk of a pressure sore? In the absence of sensation, they have to attend to everything they can in order to protect and prolong function. Christopher Reeve wrote that he was "forced to become a serious student of myself," since he had to be aware of his body all the time.[6]

"I observe objects, but not my own body." People with tetraplegia do observe their own bodies, partly because they are there in front of them, unfelt and unmoving, and so more of an object, but also because they have to, in order to protect them. Colin talked of being vigilant, and of how he tunes into what his body can tell him. He was even thankful for some pain to alert him to what might be happening. Removal of these sensations, inconstant and inconsistent though they might be, even temporarily after an epidural, was terrifying.

Murphy expressed it thus: "My former sense of embodiment remained taken for granted. . . . My sense of re-embodiment is problematic, negative and conscious. . . . Consuming consciousness of handicap even invades one's dreams."[7]

The body that one cannot feel or move, compels attention, continually and cruelly revealing itself and your new situation. What for Colin had been a source of pride, of enjoyment, of ease and of pleasure, was no longer capable of giving any of these. Previously it was through his body that he had existed in the world, in all the jobs and games. Now the body that he saw was wrecked, a visible presence reminding him constantly of his dependence and loss. His body, a symbol of his impotence, was also something he needed to care for and look after in a wholly new way. Before, he had imposed his will on his body, to run, to ride, to enjoy what it allowed him to do. He relished the communion with his physicality and with a self that existed between thought and body. In an important sense, he had existed in movement. That was all gone.

Now his body required him to care for it and think about it and protect it each day and each hour. His self had been expressed in and through his body; now that self was at the mercy of a lifeless body. Thirty years later, he remains ambivalent, knowing that he needs to nurse his body but having no pride in it and realizing that his few pleasures, of drinking and smoking, may not preserve what function he has.

Varieties of Anger

In one of his typically erudite and tortuous essays, Nick Humphrey considers faith healing and the placebo effect.[8] He develops a cogent argument, based on evolutionary principles, to explain why some people are so susceptible to healing by suggestion, or by permission of others. He quotes an experiment in which Shlomo Breznitz asked subjects to suffer pain and then altered their expectations on how long it would last. Subjects had one hand placed in painful ice-cold water and were timed as to how long they could tolerate it before they had to remove the hand. One group were told that the test would last no more than four minutes; the other was told nothing, even though the test was for four minutes in both groups. Sixty percent of the first group lasted the full four minutes, whereas only 30 percent of the second lasted that long. Knowing how long something is going to last allows one to manage one's resources.

Colin and Graham know that there will be no deliverance. Both are skeptical of a cure, even with the pace of stem cell research. This makes enduring more difficult for them. For Colin, "the only thing to look forward to is the fact that it is going to get progressively worse. To manage that is very difficult."

A consequence of this, for Colin, was—and is—an initial and prolonged anger, a rage continuing even to this day, many years after. "I could not do anything. It is a shocking situation to deal with. I do deal with it, even now thirty years later, but I cannot come to terms with it. I never come to terms. I just had too much of a life, too much to live for that no amount of counselling or patronizing could help. I got so angry, I wanted to do so much more."

This is seen in Murphy's account, too, with anger over the condition and the way it imposes, day by day, upon action and being:

Given the magnitude of this assault on the self, it is understandable that another major component of the subjective life of the handicapped is anger. . . . The anger takes two forms. The first is an existential anger, a pervasive bitterness at one's fate, a hoarse and futile cry or rage against fortune. . . . The other kind of anger is a situational one, a reaction to frustration or to what is perceived as poor treatment. . . . A paralytic may struggle to walk and become enraged when he cannot move his leg. Or a quadriplegic may pick up a cup of coffee with stiffened hands and drop it in his lap. . . . Such frustrations happen several times per day. They are minor but cumulative, and they acquire special intensity.[9]

This anger may initially focus on one's own body and its limitations, but it is also a consequence of interactions with the able-bodied world in day-to-day activities, as we will see. Whatever the problem, and whether the grievance is imagined or real, those with tetraplegia also have limited ways of expressing their frustrations. This is not simply because of their physical limitations—they can hardly storm off—but because of their fragile relations with many of those they meet. Again, in Murphy's words, "To make matters worse, as the price for normal relations, they must comfort others about their own condition. They cannot show fear, sorrow, depression, sexuality, or anger, for this disturbs the able-bodied. They cannot storm off. The unsound of limb are permitted only to laugh."[10]

One imagines that some release of feelings is possible with those close to one, but alas, for some with spinal cord injury they may have few such people at hand, and are aware that they should not try such a relationship too much. Nor is it possible, necessarily, to express these feelings within oneself. There have been debates as to whether the experience of anger is as vivid or intense in those with spinal cord injury, because it cannot be felt below the neck and embodied.[11-13] Though it is very difficult for individuals before and after spinal cord injury to be sure, those I have spoken to consider their emotional experience as intense after as before. There is, however, a sense they are aware of that they cannot dissolve into physical release of emotions to feel and dissipate them, except through voice or limited action. As Graham said, "Anger does not involve, or require, throwing something across the room. It is in the mind, and I don't think anger needs external expression. I have always tended to express it internally, otherwise it is counterproductive. . . . Anger, though, is the same."

Such a relationship between mind and body and embodied action is not solely related to expressing anger or heightened emotions. Movement falls into three types: locomotor, to navigate through the world; instrumental, the use of tools; and gesture. In addition to the feeling of the movement, all these have an aspect related to the affective or emotionally charged involvement of the subject in that movement. It is pleasurable to jog, to dance, to be connected with and to be at one with one's body. We are rarely nonaffectively involved with our bodies, rarely emotionally indifferent. Both Colin and Graham were very aware they lacked this. Graham was surprised at just how much he had enjoyed being in a tricycle with hand controls, not just for the ability to move independently, precious though that was, but also because of the sheer exhilaration of it. "One reason why I enjoy that cycling is because it is a raw physical release. Before I did not realize how badly I needed it."

Colin had never recovered from this disconnection between mind and body. As he had said, "You just cannot substitute the experience of being able to use this wonderful piece of equipment, be it running, riding, or shagging. . . . I can never forget that I am in a chair. I am devastated by my body now."

Robert Murphy made a slightly different point, that the absence of physical release into action robs the tetraplegic not only of that pleasurable aspect of movement but also of the merging of mind and body that sometimes occur during movement, with thoughts anchored in place and time more leadenly: "A quadriplegic's body can no longer speak a 'silent language.' . . . The thinking activity can no longer be dissolved into motion, and the mind can no longer be lost in an internal dialogue with physical movement."[14]

Just as one has to become less spontaneous with spinal cord injury—and many other impairments—planning movements and using them efficiently, so in one's thoughts spontaneity and even imagination may be affected. Without this ease of action and of movement, and without independence and easy interaction with others, Graham and Colin agreed that spinal cord injury became all-pervasive in their dreams and their daytime thoughts. Robert Murphy pointed out that "consciousness is overtaken and devoured in contemplation, meditation, ratiocination, and reflection without end, relieved only by one's remaining movements and sleep. . . . My thoughts and sense of being alive have been driven back into my brain, where I now reside. More than ever it is the base from which I reach out and grasp the world. . . . Many say they are no longer attached to their bodies."[15]

For all three of them this driving back into the brain was associated with an altered relationship and view of their bodies. Murphy wrote of an emotional detachment from his body, "*the* leg, *the* arm," rather than his leg and arm. Colin could not accept his body as it was: "I was proud of my physical stature when I was young and fit. Now I have not come to terms with my body. Can you accept that this is your lot and you have to make your new life? I cannot." For Colin, however, unlike Robert Murphy, this inaction did not lead to a disassociation from his body. One huge aspect of Colin's life that he finds so difficult to talk about, and only volunteered in response to a direct question, is pain. This we will return to later, but he was quite clear that he would prefer pain to having no sensation at all, because pain alerts him to problems, and anchors him in his body.

Fatigue

Though one might imagine that without action one might not become tired, it seemed that, paradoxically, the absence of movement led to a great feeling of tiredness, both physical and mental. Murphy wrote, "I have been overtaken by a profound and deepening sense of tiredness [which is both physical and mental]. There is another aspect of tiredness which cannot be cured by rest . . . a sense of tiredness and ennui with practically everything and everybody, a desire to withdraw from the world . . . sometimes because they are depressed, but more often because they must each day face an inimical world."[16]

Graham agreed. During his physiotherapy, he was tired by the increasing physical demands, but also he had noticed that the injury causes tiredness in itself. Sitting in a chair might be considered a passive and easy thing to do; but those who live in a chair often have problems holding their head up with weakened neck muscles, and with balancing as best they can in the chair without postural trunk movement. They take visual fixes from a spot on the wall opposite to keep their relation with the chair and the floor constant, just as pirouetting ballerinas take spots to keep their balance. Tetraplegics balance in their chairs for hours each day. This may be tiring enough, but there is also a suggestion that spinal cord injury leads to chronic tiredness of itself.

Four Changes in Consciousness

By being unable, even for a short time, to forget they were in a chair and were tetraplegic, spinal cord injury affects consciousness. Murphy thought the four most far-reaching changes in the consciousness of the disabled were a lowered self-esteem, the invasion and occupation of thought by physical deficits, a strong undercurrent of anger, and the acquisition of a new, total, and undesirable identity. One consequence of these was a shrinking of the world and a turning in on oneself. He describes people with quadriplegia who stayed at home, half blaming society but also half knowing the withdrawal to be their own fault.

"Our lives are built upon a constant struggle between the need to reach out to others and a contrary urge to fall back into ourselves." He described "one man never going out and no one ever visiting, even his children's friends. . . . There is a balance between the falling back into ourselves and a need to reach out. . . . Amongst the disabled the inward pull becomes compelling, often irresistible."[17]

Graham and Colin denied that their injuries had had this effect. Both worked and had a sense of purpose after their injury. I sensed that their balance between withdrawal and outward looking had not been tilted at the time of their injury and when working, but that it might have been, more recently, years after their injury. To work and live independently was, after all, nearly a full-time occupation with tetraplegia. The maintenance of a social life as well could be too much, especially as one became older. Colin suggested this and had decided to work to secure financial independence later. For both it was as though the years of trying so hard to be outward looking had taken their toll; Colin was content to spend some of his spare time relatively solitarily. More recently, and after I had spoken with him, he told me that he had taken early retirement.[18]

Happy Days?

Robert Murphy documented the consequences his physical loss had on his esteem and selfhood:

The totality of the impact of serious physical impairment on conscious thought . . . gives disability a far stronger purchase on one's sense of who and what he is than do any social roles . . . which can be manipulated. Each social role can be adjusted to the audience, each role played before a separate audience, allowing us to lead multiple lives. One cannot however shelve a disability or hide it. . . . It is not a role; it is an identity. . . . Society will not let him forget it.[19]

The physical loss is an impairment not only of mobility and sensation but almost of consciousness and selfhood itself. The roles we adopt and play with others, which are part of the social interactions we enjoy and explore, become limited, related to and grounded in the chair, dependent on people's reduced expectations. Thus Colin said that he could never forget that he was in a chair, never become engrossed in a book or film, and never escape from his limitations.

One might think that the days of Graham and Colin were filled with an indefinable undercurrent of anger; talking with them, this was obviously not the case, and it may have been overemphasized during our conversation. But when I raised their enjoyment of more positive motions such as laughter and joy, they were measured in their responses.[20]

It was as though, even though humor was not banished, the injury had so tilted their view of the world, and of other people and other situations, that they saw funny in the distance, as something happening to others. It was less that anger threatened to take over and suffocate other, more positive, feelings; it was that their situation was such that they could not reach out to others through the comic, or take fun from others into themselves, or disarm some of the mild setbacks in life that we all have with humour.

According to Colin, "I can see humor in the world, but—and I know it sounds very self-centered—but I am so angry and bitter at having the pleasures of the world taken from me at such an early age."

Similarly, Graham had said that he could not claim to have ever been happy or content since he was in a wheelchair. "For me each day life is either bearable or unbearable. It has never really got beyond that. How did I come to terms with it? I just did. . . . Since I have been disabled, I cannot claim that I have ever been happy. It is too much a struggle, every day."

For each day to be bearable or not. . . . Samuel Beckett used losses of embodiment to approach the areas in which he was interested between being and not being. It is therefore not surprising that several times he deprived his characters of movement. In his play *Happy Days*,[21] Winnie spends the first act living up to her waist in sand and the second up to her neck. The parallels with spinal injury are clear. For Winnie, happy days are ones when she sees someone, or when her husband and carer speak to her—social, interpersonal events.

In Beckett's novel *Murphy*, the eponymous hero, who finds work and much social interaction beyond him, seeks solace by withdrawing from his body, by sitting in a rocking chair, naked, slowing down all movement to release his mind: "He sat in his chair in this way because it gave him pleasure! First it gave his body pleasure, it appeased his mind. Then it set him free in his mind. For it was not until his body was appeased that he could come alive in his mind. . . . And life in his mind gave him pleasure, such pleasure that pleasure was not the word."[22]

Here, however, there was an element of choice, and his apparent freedom from his body was pleasurable and temporary, so different from the experiences of those with spinal injury. In the final of Beckett's great trilogy of novels, *The Unnamable*, the narrator, without name or identity, spends his days—without movement or feeling—within a jar or container, engaged in what appears to be an internal monologue.

All that is left to the narrator are thoughts and words; silence is the ultimate negation. His monologue is a meditation on existence under those conditions and, by extension, under all conditions. "Notice, I notice nothing, I go on as best I can, if it begins to mean something I can't help it." In the last parts of the book, his thoughts and words, all that he has and is, keep silence (his life's end) away. Several times he echoes, "You must go on, I can't go on, I'll go on."[23]

Beckett's work has similarities with that of another writer, from another age and another place:

> Only some of the people behave in this way. The others are not going anywhere: they have nowhere to go, and no reason to go there. They drift this way and that, sit in the shade, stare, nap. They have nothing to do. No one is expecting them. . . . For they are everywhere around here, idle, awaiting who knows what, living who knows how—the gapers of the world. . . .
> They will not return to the countryside, and there is no place in the city. They endure. Somehow they exist. Somehow; that is how best to describe their situation, its fragility, its uncertainty. Somehow one lives, somehow one sleeps, somehow.[24]

The others Ryszard Kapuscinski describes are those millions of Africans who migrate to cities without money, work, or a place to stay. They too endure at the margins, not because of illness—though that arrives all too soon—but because of poverty and a lack of connection with the society they gawp at. Life, however meager, is endured, without question or complaint.

To endure: to suffer without resistance, to exist without giving way. Beckett would, I think, have recognized Graham saying that "each day life is either bearable or unbearable. It has never really got beyond that."

The experiences of Graham and Colin are similar in their spinal level and in responses. Yet it always seems odd to say to a person with, say, diabetes, "Come over here, there is another diabetic, you will have lots to talk about." Why define a person solely by their impairment? The consequences of spinal cord injury may impose common problems on those who live with the condition but, equally well, there will be individuals whose responses to those problems are very different and whose lives have different relationships to their injuries.

In the next chapters we follow those with different experiences and very different views on the nature of endurance with tetraplegia. Some have continued their lives with a minimum of disruption and with no anguish or anger; others have denied that anger and, instead, sought to alter societies' view of their impairment. But before these we will consider, in the next two chapters, two men whose views and relationships to their injuries have changed hugely, from indifference to despair, and then to accommodation as they have moved on.

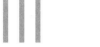

Exploring

5

Heads Up to the World

Words of Encouragement

David was a big man, even in a chair. Knowing of my arrival, he had read a previous book of mine to see where I was coming from.[1] I hoped this was a good omen. We chatted over coffee before he started to talk about the moment it began.

"I broke my neck in a diving accident, running in off the beach into the sea and not breaking the water cleanly with my hands, taking all the impact on the point of my chin, pushing my head backwards and breaking my neck. The only thing I could do was lie face down in the water. I could feel nothing at all, and I could move my neck about half an inch sideways each way. The rest of me was in spinal shock. My friends realized that I was laying flat down in the water and not playing around, so they got me out. At the moment they got me clear of the water, I said, 'Mind my head because I have broken my neck.' I just intuitively knew. I had no idea what it meant for the rest of my life, but I knew what I had done."

David was taken via the local ER to a neurosurgical ward. He had a respiratory arrest the first night in the hospital and was in intensive care for six weeks. After five months, he was transferred to the local spinal unit, where he spent the next year. He was twenty-one and had just finished a university degree in chemistry. That summer holiday was to have been the last time he and his friends played together before they went their separate ways.

From the start David's attitude was enquiring.

"I was conscious for all of it, apart from the respiratory arrest. I was concerned with the practicalities, I suppose, of getting on with life. I didn't lie there thinking all the time, 'Oh my God, what have I done, what's this going to mean?' I never burst into tears because, from the early stages of living with the injury, I have seen the whole thing as a challenge. How do I overcome so and so? How do I deal with this? How do I come to terms with that? I never thought, 'I can't do that.'"

His first thoughts and hopes were of recovery. That option slid slowly away from him with the weeks.

"I would have liked to have been told fairly soon because it would have enabled me to get a clearer focus on things. It was allowed to just seep in as I found myself moved from a neurosurgical ward in a district hospital to a spinal unit, and then on meeting up with other people in similar stages as your own. Guys came in for checkups who had been injured years ago, and I could see that's what I was going to be like if I was lucky. I saw paras and tetras. Every tetraplegic dreams of being a paraplegic."

He had several operations to stabilize his neck, and then he was allowed to sit up, which allowed him to begin to feed himself—a really important thing after several weeks of lying on his back totally dependent. Then, after learning to get out of bed without fainting, it was occupational therapy and physiotherapy. His goals in movement were small and achievable; these kept out the bigger questions, at least for a while. In the United Kingdom thirty years ago, there was no counselling. The health care professionals might look after his physical problems and pass the time of day, but they were not really able to go deeper. That probably suited David at the time; he had never considered discussing feelings professionally.

"Most of my learning about me, my injury and the effect it was going to have on me, was done through fellow patients going through the same thing."

He ended up with a C5/6 complete tetraplegia. He can flex his elbows, extend his wrists, and turn his forearms over, but he has no finger movement. From the chest down, he is completely paralyzed; below that level he can feel odd patches of sensation that vary from time to time. He cannot feel his bladder and bowels as such, but he does have some feeling he interprets as fullness. There has been no change in the last thirty years.

At the spinal unit he was told to, "get on with the rest of your life, because in twenty years you are going to be dead." It was made clear that he would die from a chest or urine infection, or from pressure sores. "One of those would kill you in twenty years, guaranteed," was the message we got. The head of unit put it that starkly in those days. But it was done in an encouraging fashion. What it meant was, "Get on and live your life, and don't hang around for things, because you won't have the life span other people have."

When he came out of hospital after seventeen months, in December 1972, his options were twofold. Either he went straight into a charitably run home for the chronically disabled, or he went back to live with his family. His father managed a straight job swap, and his parents moved to the West Country from Suffolk to look after him.

Before his injury David had had a job in engineering in Birmingham on a graduate management-training scheme. He had been due to go on their training course, rotating through the different departments. They held the job open for twelve months, but then he had to admit he could not take it up. Instead he found work at the university Stationery Office. Six months later, having proved he could work full time, he moved to a firm of insurance brokers. He ended up working there for ten years, while living at home. In the early seventies, it was difficult for someone in a wheelchair to find employment, so he was really pleased. The job was not just about money; it gave him independence and, he says quite simply, a reason for being. It was more important for him than for most of his able-bodied colleagues.

"At work the only concession was that I slipped off work quarter of an hour early to miss the rush hour. I used to get home, crash out for an hour, get up, have a bite to eat, and go out for the evening. As a twenty-two or twenty-three year old, you have the energy. Friends, cinema, pubs, I was accused of treating home like a hotel, which I think, secretly, my parents were really quite pleased with."

He did his professional insurance exams by correspondence courses over three years and passed the first time. He swam for a club of disabled people. Friends thought he was crazy because he had broken his neck swimming, but for ten years he rushed thrashing up and down the pool, enjoying the competition. He lived life to the full, to his full.

Then he began to have problems with his neck. A wire loop that had been inserted to stabilize his neck had slowly acted like a cheese cutter, paring through the neck to push onto the spinal cord. Over the next eighteen months he had three operations to remove the wire and restabilize the neck. Having spent a decade ignoring his injury as best he could, this was a jarring return to dependency and illness. After the surgery, he took early retirement on health grounds.

Time Expired

For the next seven or eight years, David lived at home. He had little to say about this time. Slowly he realized that the end of his twenty-year lifespan was coming closer and that he was living on borrowed time. Though confiding in no one, he began to wait for the bad chest infection or the urine infection, and slowly, his mood drifted down. Then there were several illnesses, eventually found to be related to a hormonal imbalance that was only diagnosed when he went into a coma.[2] By then, ill and worried that his time was up, he would have accepted not waking up the next day. He had not previously considered suicide and still would not have considered actively ending his life, but a painless slip into oblivion, with no recriminations from family and friends, had its appeal.

"I was not well and did not know what was the matter with me. Nobody else did, either. I was getting fatter and fatter and more bloated. Every day was a struggle, and with this physical illness I began not to like myself at all. Now I can look in the mirror and say, 'Well you are all right, and I like you.' But then, I didn't. I really hated myself. Things had gradually crept up on me. I had been well for over twenty years after my injury, beyond my projected lifespan."

Previously he had constructed a life full of friends and family, and one almost independent of his injury. Now he saw himself in purely physical terms, dependent and sick. Life, he thought, had passed him by, with no relationships beyond his family, and no family of his own. He had wasted half his projected span, since giving up work, and now that time was nearly over.

"I was in hospital over one New Year period, came out, and was still recovering. Lying in bed at my folks' home, I caught myself thinking, 'What am I doing, why am I lying here with my face to the wall just waiting to die?'"

David had passed over this period when we first met. On a subsequent visit, he discussed this period of depression with some objectivity. He mentioned how reading a book on depression by Dorothy Rowe had helped him, and he loaned it to me.[3] He had underlined the relevant passages. At home, as I read, I could well imagine the solace the words gave, showing him he was not alone. But as I read, I was struck again and again about how apposite Rowe's words on depression were to some with spinal cord injury: "It is not simply loneliness. . . . It is an isolation which changes your perception of your environment. Intellectually you know you are sharing a space with other people . . . but even though you can reach out and touch another . . . nothing is transmitted. Even objects around you seem further away."

Living from a wheelchair may well alter one's perception of the world and of one's movement within it. Without touch and tactile exploration of the world, things may appear further away, one's lived space may be reduced.

"How can you describe this experience and convey its meaning to someone else. . . . The turmoil of your feelings is so great that it is impossible to know where to begin to describe them. So it is better to remain silent."

David had always looked forwards and outwards. But now, with the passing of his expected lifespan, he began to look inside to feelings he could hardly understand or articulate. Expressing feelings was, after all, not what men of his generation did.

The most elaborate images are those where the person finds himself trapped: an endless tunnel, a cold dungeon, sealed in a metal sphere or a black balloon. Cages come in many shapes and sizes: a diving bell or abandoned high on a Ferris wheel . . . however the image is expressed, all images have one thing in common. The person is enduring a terrible isolation.

If you told people how frightened you are they would think you mad. . . . The fear is so great that death might be welcome as peace, a cessation of the fear. . . . The fear permeates your life; undermining your confidence. . . . Sometimes the fear comes . . . in the special guise of guilt. . . . You have failed yourself and other people. You have not lived up to the expectations of yourself. . . . Death may bring peace, but it will take away the hope that one day the terrible grief you bear will be recompensed. . . . You tell no one of this. . . .

Now no one needs you, no one admires or respects you. You fear being dependent on others and having them pity you. Or are you mourning a dream, something that was once bright and splendid but now unrealisable in this hard, cruel and sordid world? There will be no promised land, no happy ending. Such losses are hard to name and even harder to mourn. . . .

Once you were ambitious: now you are bitterly resigned to your awful fate and cannot fight against it. You are filled with grey and heavy indifference, even towards people who were once important to you. Love has fled, leaving only an awareness of the absence of love. You do not love, but you are filled with bitterness and jealousy. Bitter that your life has gone awry and jealous that other people, quite undeserving, have such easy lives and do not suffer as you do. You hate yourself for feeling such horrendous jealousy, just as you hate yourself for being unable to love (pp. 4–8).

These words underlined by David were written about depression, but mirrored his view of his own time-expired life. David had never previously asked the questions, "What if?" and "Why me?" This was not through any conscious effort; it was just the way he was. Each problem had been faced, each viewed as something to be overcome as best he could. Now the doubts emerged. Even after the years of successful working and enjoying life to the full, he began to question its validity, to question his validity. Rowe again was underlined:

You can never be the person you think you ought to be, or achieve the things you feel you ought to achieve. You may believe that your luck has run out. . . . You will leave behind no work that you will be remembered by: your virtues will not be extolled, you leave no children behind you to revere you. When you die you will be forgotten. It will be as if you never existed.

Rowe went on to suggest ways of recovering and escaping from the despair, but David had not underlined these.

Flipping a Coin

He knew he needed professional help. Though he had never considered therapy before, and indeed had not been sympathetic to such an approach, he contacted the clinical psychologist at his local spinal treatment center. Over the next fifteen months, he saw the psychologist, Rob, for an hour once every two weeks, travelling the fifty miles or so there and back each time. During each hour, David would talk for fifty-five minutes or more, pouring out his feelings of uselessness. For fifteen months, this was the most important part of his life. Rob did not tell him what to do, could not provide answers, but rather allowed David to find his own solution as best he could.

"What I needed when I first met him was to unburden myself completely. I could not hold back. That was so hard."

David had told no one of his fears, thinking the best way was not to express, not to explore feelings. His hopes previously had required silence, and for the first twenty years or so, that had pretty much worked. The psychologist supported David and showed him ways out of his depression. But one important fact Rob did tell David: advances in medical care meant that his lifespan was not limited to twenty years at all. Though, by then, David had problems over and above this, the fact that he was not out of time was hugely welcome. David began to explore new ideas, new feelings, and new ways of living.

"We would address a new problem every couple of weeks. It worked brilliantly for me and turned my whole approach to life over, like flipping a coin. Instead of being head down to the world, I was head up and getting on with things."

Afterwards David was so fascinated he enrolled in a course in psychology and for an introductory course in counselling before deciding they were not for him.

"I've always thought in logical terms, and I didn't have a great deal of time for airy fairy things like, as I saw, counselling. My experience with Rob has completely turned that around. Now I am probably the most open to all sorts of different ideas, ways of doing things, different aspects, and personalities, open as a person more than I have ever been."

David even took a course in English literature, to learn more about people and their relationships, to express himself better, and to understand the emotions being portrayed by playwrights or authors. He studied Shakespeare, Ibsen, Browning, and Dickens. He turned from a pure scientist, rejoicing in the rules and laws of natural science, to someone keen to understand the messy and unpredictable slop of normal human existence. It also meant that he had to go to college and study with others. Seeing his tetraplegia, some people suggested distance learning might be easier. But he needed to get out and see people again. Time with others was as therapeutic as the study.

His depression was due to a combination of things: his acute illness, his erroneous perception that he had exceeded his lifespan, and a slower realization of what the injury involved. But there was also a more acute problem: his parents were aging and he knew that he might find himself in a long-term home, "for the young disabled," when they found themselves unable to cope.

Rob suggested a completely novel idea: might he live on his own? For David, unable to move more than his upper arms and who had lived with his parents since his injury, such an idea was unimaginable. He did not dismiss it, though it was several months later that he rang the local independent living scheme.

Letting Go

The problems of moving out were huge. He had to find a place and several full-time carers, and manage them himself. He had to find furniture, somewhere that could be adapted for him, hoists, and a gardener. But, restored once more, he now viewed these as challenges.

If moving into a new place was one problem, leaving his parents was another. They had spent the last eighteen years or so looking after him, giving him the freedom to enjoy his youth and then, for the last eight years, supporting his "retirement." He was unsure if he had outstayed his welcome or whether they might like some time back. In the end it was both.

Fortunately there was a local center for inclusive living that helped him. Within a few months he had his own place.

"It worked absolutely brilliantly. I wouldn't go back now. It can be hard work but it's really worthwhile doing and it's enabled me to do all sorts of new things rather than be constrained within family ties."

David has one full-time live-in personal assistant, or PA, and three part-timers, all on proper contracts. David does it all himself despite the work, becoming an expert on payroll, time sheets, budgeting, and the law (European Working Time Directive, Stakeholder Pensions, etc.). He receives money into his bank accounts from the local authority and from the government-run Independent Living Fund. Despite being relatively costly, by passing the running over to the user and not needing local care homes, it works out cheaper for the government.

"I appreciate being completely in control of my own circumstances and employ someone as an assistant, doing the things I can't do for myself in day-to-day living. They don't *care* for me at all."

I searched for an analogy and suggested that maybe for a carer, as opposed to a PA, looking after someone suggested almost a mother/child relationship, in which one side did not simply care but might also control. David agreed. "Very much so—and I think that's a good analogy—mother/child relationship as in a carer. It could easily become like that. A carer would not work for me very long before I would find all sorts of things I did not want. They might mean well, but I would be doing what they wanted. I need to say when anything is done, how it's done, and the way it's done."

An increasing problem is recruitment; people can get jobs in supermarkets for the same money. He advertises in various magazines and on the net. He prefers Scandinavians because they are familiar with the PA/carer divide. On cue, Anneca, his present PA, walked in. She was in her late twenties, with a ready, deep, smile.

"I liked David's personal way of putting his advert and the way everything was carried out professionally. When people ask what I do, I say I do the things for him he can't do for himself. Luckily, he is very articulate and can easily direct his PAs, so he can make things happen in the way he wants."

These matters may seem simple, even trivial, but are quite the opposite. Normally we decide to move— to have a cup of tea or go out—and we do it. Action follows intention, and we have no problem with ascribing that action as being ours. But what if our intentions are delayed or altered? Then our sense of the action being our own fades. Those with spinal cord injury need to feel a direct relation between intention and action, to feel in control of what happens, even though they need someone else to make the action happen.

Anneca said she knew if she took the job, David had something to offer in exchange. He has helped her with the language and with taking several part-time courses. David continued, "I encourage anybody who comes to live in as a PA to develop their own interests so they are not entirely bound up with me. You start off with an employer/employee relationship. By the end, you end up being companionable, though it's not until somebody finishes that you might call him or her a friend. I have that difference in my own mind."

Anneca agreed. "David is very good at distinguishing between private life and professional. He would only ask for anything out of hours if it was urgent. Sometimes I find him struggling on his own because he won't take advantage of my time, and I really appreciate that. I don't feel like I have to escape the house the minute I clock off, and I can easily stay here twenty-four hours without feeling trapped."

Much of David's time can be spent recruiting PAs.

"I realized I've got to recruit regularly, yearly. Anneca came for six months and is going after eighteen. I'm about to see who turns up next. To begin with, I found it quite scary. Now, because I'm on top of things, I find it slightly more interesting; it's always nice to see who turns up. I prefer women, mainly because they are better around the house. I am aware of the need to be very welcoming, very open, and very clear about what I want. When they start, I say this must be a lot scarier for you than it is for me. I am used to this changeover but for you this is a major step. What can I do to help you settle in?"

David is so at home and in control that one does not question his independence at all. On leaving home he was very careful not to lose his relationship with his parents, and initially he called them twice a day without fail. He was delighted that with their new free time his parents took some holidays and started going out to the theater and doing amateur dramatics again. They rejoiced in their newfound independence, just as he did, with neither side feeling bereft.

Matters of Fact

Anneca left, and I asked what he needed for day-to-day care. He had a hoist for transfers and a set of portable ramps. Once in bed, though, he was "like a fish out of water." Being so tall he had help with dressing, though he does wash and do his own teeth. He has had an indwelling urinary catheter for ten years or so. He had used continual intermittent drainage before, but found he was having bladder infections. Bowels were a problem about five percent of the time.

"They are part of my daily routine, and I take my PAs on a training course. Manual evacuation is so quick—just two minutes. New staff see it as a hurdle to get over, but I treat it as very matter of fact."

He made it all sound so easy—and of course it is when approached so sensibly. I moved on to enquire about the sensations he lived with. He said he lives with pain, mainly in the back, but that it is not severe and requires no medication.

"Very occasionally I can feel my toes, but couldn't tell you which, though I could tell you which foot. I also have odd patches of sensation below my level, so I feel 95 percent complete. Sensation may not come through the cord but through the parasympathetic system.[4] I use these terms because I have always been fascinated in what is happening to my own body."

He quite likes some pain because it makes him feel connected with his body.

"If it was a complete cut off, absolutely nothing, it would be really weird. If I sleep with my arm outside the covers and cut the blood supply off and I have a dead arm—then it is total different from the way I feel with the bit of feeling that I have. Numbness is definitely something. The pain, while it might be localized, does actually give me a semblance of my lower half. I don't like it when it's nagging away, but it would be very strange to be without any feeling whatsoever below the level of my lesion. You could stick a needle into me and I wouldn't have any idea, but I feel the pain as being there in the legs.[5]

"I've got so used to moving my legs around and touching them that it doesn't strike me as at all odd that I can't feel my leg. If I move my leg slightly, I have movement sensations up through into my back, and I can feel it around the back and neck level. I can be touched and not feel that, but from a little bit of movement, then I know."

David showed me what he calls his "saving grace." He took a drink, and as he extended his wrist back toward him so his fingers flexed, due to contraction of the tendons that normally straighten the fingers, and this produced an artificial grip. "I let them contract just about the right amount for me." As he reached forward for the drink, the effort to avoid falling was obvious.

"When I was first in hospital, I did all sorts of balancing exercises. My balance was appalling to begin with, but years and years on it's a lot better, so I can close my eyes and move my limbs around and know where my arms are in space. It took a while to explore that; you learn to balance with all the muscles you've got and you build up a body map."

But this is a body map with no movement below the elbows and no reliable sensation below the thumbs. The muscles he could use in the arm were weak, and he had none in the trunk. Sitting in a chair was not an easy option.

Living in the Head

The book of mine that David had read was on the effects of facial difference. One chapter concerned James, a man born without facial expression. David picked out several sentences from this chapter.

I have a notion which has stayed with me over much of my life. That it's possible to live in your head, entirely in my head. . . . I had feelings of low self esteem and loneliness and isolation in company. . . . If you say where does me now reside I think I am slowly coming out of my head a bit. I am not sure I can locate where I am but I don't think I'm entirely in my head or even my mind. . . . I have an expression of living a life of the mind but I do accept the mind is not easily able to communicate its thoughts or even its feelings or I suppressed a lot of them and I have been told I am a very placid person.[6]

David continued, "Much resonated with me about living in your head. I am a very placid person. Nothing to do with my injury, I've always been like it. So I miss out, and I am aware I miss out, on the whole range of emotions. One of the things I am doing now is using body language, naturally, to increase my expressiveness. That's getting better as I'm getting older. I am much more happy to allow myself to be swayed by emotion, to sit and cry in front of people."

James, I had suggested, without emotion on his face, found it difficult to show emotion through gesture or voice as well. Without face, the other channels for expression might not have been so developed. I had encouraged him to inhabit his body expressively, not least because once you communicate with others you get something back. Some had suggested that people with tetraplegia might have less emotional experience, as we have seen. David was aware of these matters.

"I do gesticulate a lot, though I don't normally think about it. I can't move much, so the bits I can move, I move a lot more to help me emphasize points." He was also helped because he had not lost his deep, commanding voice. He went back to James. I had suggested to him that in discussing his sense of self and where it resided, it seemed that the more it might reside in his body, and in his arms, rather than in his head, then the closer he might be to the world and to others. David had also picked this out. "I agree. I am aware of this living in the head because the rest of my body does not work very well, if at all. I identify with James' feeling that 'If I can be more in my body I would feel more part of the world.'"

David, unlike James, had more than an emotional limit in movement.

"I like to be doing things physically, I feel much more engaged with whatever is happening around. If I sit and read, or think or just talk, then in a way it's not enough. I need to be doing things physically for them to mean that little bit more. The 'me,' as in 'Where am I, my inner self,' I would like to drag more out of my head into my body. But I am limited by how much physically my body will move and how much sensation I've got. I would like to spread it out more, but I can't."

He said this as fact, not tragedy.

"Part of this is how I see me, and part of it is also how others perceive me. My wheelchair, for instance, is not part of me. It might need to fit me like a pair of trousers; it might need to be there when I want it to do what I want to do, but it is not part of me. The frustrating thing is that the chair itself, any wheelchair, acts as a barrier between others and me. When people see me, they see the chair first."

"When on top of things, I am pretty good at making sure people talk to me, listen to me, and react with me, rather than take notice of the chair. But the chair does get in the way physically. I have sat in an easy chair in the past, but it's not particularly comfortable, and I would be concerned about the effects on my backside."

No Magic Wand

David's days are full. Having worked full time for ten years, he has a small pension, which, with his Disability Living allowance, is enough to live on. He has no desire to be in an office again. He does a huge amount of voluntary work as an assessor for the Social Services Inspectorate, looking at independent living for disabled people. He has spent some time writing a user guidebook for independent living. But helping others, putting back what he took out, is only one part of his life. Like his parents, he loves theatre. He has been traveling as much as he feels able. He was amazed at how accessible Prague was, and how advanced facilities are in Sweden. In Stockholm, he even got on and off the underground without any problem, a far cry from London. Still, each trip is a challenge, from planning to doing.

In Copenhagen, he checked into a hotel with his PA and his brother and decided to go for a stroll on his own, arranging to meet later at the Tivoli Gardens. For an hour or so he just wandered around in his electric wheelchair. The idea of being alone on a street in a foreign capital would have been unimaginable a few years earlier. He also likes risk. He goes down escalators front ways, with somebody holding on the back as best they can. He has recently taken up ultralight flying.

"Partly because your opportunities for an adrenalin rush are so limited, I like to put myself in these situations. Having been right at the edge, nearly dead already, there is that fascination to explore that edge again. It is also because the opportunities for things like relationships are reduced. The rush from feeling head over heels in love with somebody is gone."

I was surprised, because I had not thought that people went into relationships for that rush.

"No, but that's one of the things you can get from it. I can remember last time I was in love, before the injury. It was like a hammer thumping away in your chest."

I wondered if some of a tetraplegic's "reduced emotional experience" might come from lack of opportunity. Christopher Reeve has talked of the "numb zone" when nothing is happening. David agreed.

"I would describe myself now as heads up to the world. Some people have said being injured was one of the best things that ever happened to them. I wouldn't agree, but I would say that I am quite comfortable being me. I can understand now what these people are talking about. Since I have been injured, I have met some absolutely wonderful people. If you've got good friends and family around you, it makes life a lot easier. Over the last few years, particularly since I have moved in here managing entirely by myself, I'm comfortable with who I am.

"There are all sorts of things in life that I miss, but they tend to be relatively minor. I don't miss being able to walk or run around. I have not missed it for a long, long time. What I do miss are the little things, feeling the springiness of grass under your feet, or feeling the squelch of mud between your toes. I miss being able to make music. Piano was the most expressive way of getting my emotions out. I miss being in control of the instrument, the coordination to play, the pleasure of constructing the movements. You move into things like muscle memory; how is it you learn notes and then phrases, and suddenly you see a phrase and you play a phrase, not an individual note? For years after my injury, maybe up to the first five years, it bugged me that I could not play anything."

Now he is content to hear others play; perhaps it is not coincidence that most of his PAs have played an instrument. As we chatted, Anneca was in her room, practicing her violin, filling the house with the sounds of Bach as her fingers moved over the strings. I asked if, given the chance, he would return to full movement and sensation. He thought for a moment.

"Why might I not? Why might I not want to? Well, I think thirty years down the line I am used to being who I am. I would actually have to go through a grieving process for losing me as I am now. That would be very strange. I could work my way through it, but it might come across as negating all the love and friendship as a result of being spinally injured. Putting that to one side and saying I was moving onto another phase in my life would be difficult. Because I am as happy as I am, I don't really feel the need to want to change. Lastly, the logic in me actually says that I would never recover enough to make it worthwhile. You can't wave a magic wand."

I offered him a theoretical wand.

"Even then I don't know. It's been a struggle to get to where I am now—all sorts of hurdles along the way which I have achieved or fallen at or been helped over—but I'm pretty happy with who I am. I don't really feel the need to change, be it by magic or not."

Sitting with him in his house, talking, enjoying lunch, and now listening to Anneca playing, I had begun to enter his world, and maybe could begin to understand. David had changed in many ways over the last years. Once a chemist, now he was a student of the humanities. For many years he had ignored his spinal injury as much as possible and carried on as best he could, before being forced to confront and explore it. Since then, he had become stronger and more reconciled and set up his own home independently. As I left, Anneca came out to take our photograph. I felt a great warmth, seeing them laughing together as I got into my car.

6

Being Someone Else

A Lump of Ham

"The first thing I assessed once I came around from the operation was what I could no longer do. What the future did not hold for me. You see others in rehab, some walking, some in chairs, and you are totally self-obsessed at the beginning. I will not raise a family; I will not be independent. Someone else will have to do my bowel care, put me to bed and wash me."

In May 2000 when in his twenties, Ian had a spinal abscess. He walked into the hospital, but unfortunately, when they operated to relieve the pressure on his neck, the spinal cord suffered and he was left tetraplegic. The fact that he had not driven his car off the road or fallen drunk down stairs made it even more difficult. When I met him, still in the hospital, he had struggled with it for a year. He had also altered his views of both himself and of others in ways he could not have considered.

"As I go through it, I begin to realize that to some extent I am lucky. I am tetraplegic, C7, but with some hand movement, so I can do many things myself. I have a little sensation and so am incomplete. There is some sensation on the chest and some on the outside two toes of my right foot. Recently some has come back over the inside of my calf. Unfortunately, most of the return has been pain. If I scratch my calf, it hurts. There are other bits: to manage my bladder I use intermittent catheterization, and I can feel, very much, when I withdraw the catheter. It is painful, and that is good. Before it was completely numb. These are manageable and confirm I am alive."

"Recently I began to move my toes. It does not mean anything, and it does not mean that I am going to walk. All it suggests is that one or two nerve cells are working. But it connects me to my body, and it is nice to be able to do it. It is similar to being in a standing frame. It is nice to be in, and good to look down on something—I had forgotten how tall I was. They say it is good for bone density. But it is also nice that the physiotherapists and the other guys can see how tall I am."

"I was a contracting electrician, crawling through roof spaces every day, driving myself to work. I did not have to ask for help from anyone. I never prided myself on this; it was just what happened during the course of a day. All this has gone now."

"I lie in bed at night thinking of what has happened. These are the most difficult times, these are the times when I feel like someone else because the parameters have changed. I am now thinking in a much more limited perspective. I no longer think, 'Well, I wish I could do that,' because I know I can't. I know it will upset me. That's not to say I have given up on recovery, but I know it is unlikely, and so I do the best I can. When I touch my legs, when I am on the bed and I lift my legs with my arms and I see it is my leg, I can only feel it in the sense that when I alter the position my balance changes. It's like picking up a lump of ham. It is almost impersonal."

"My past pride in my body I let go. I cannot control my abdominal muscles, so they bulge out, and I look like a little Buddha. That bothers me a lot. I have changed shape physically. That worries me. I do intend to get fit, and I do look at the body shapes of others in chairs. It is now just me, that shape. But when I see a reflection of me in a mirror, it is not me."

"I am as a baby. Not just the physical help that is needed, but also the way I think. I need help to do so much that I have to ask for help the whole time. It all comes back to being independent. Emotionally too it is the same. I get really angry very quickly. Even with kindness when people open doors. I keep telling my mother, 'If I need help I will ask.' My stepfather tries to push me everywhere, and that is rather dangerous, since if he hits something I will fly out. I want to be independent. I have surprisingly found that I have more pride left than I thought. I had thought that my ego had collapsed, what with bowel care and being woken at night to be turned, being totally dependent on others."

A Different World with Different Rules

I wondered if there was any way he could dissociate himself from some of the things that had to be done for him, like the bowel care?

"What I can see is important, like my spasms. They used to throw me out of bed, or out of the chair, and now I have a baclofen pump, which helps a lot.[1] The worst times were when the nurses put me to bed and my legs spasm up and hit them. I hit the nurses, but it was not me who did it, and they say, 'Are you sure you don't mean to do that?' But it was not directed, not me.

"Watching your legs in spasm when you have no control, like someone else is doing it, whether you try and try or not—and I do try and there is a slight tingle down there at times—watching your legs do that is really peculiar. I recognize them as my legs, but I cannot control them. With my bowels I cannot say it is not me. Facing the other way and not being able to see what is going on is one thing but still awful. Now I am doing my own bowel care. I use a mirror, a rearview mirror, and I am still connected because I see. It is also me in control.

"I used to get dreams, bad dreams, and they have stopped now at last. I was in my chair at a football match one Sunday and the kids would be kicking the ball and it would come towards me and I would try to get up to kick it, feel a jolt, and try to get up and could not, and wake up. That same thing would occur in other situations. I used to be in the merchant navy, and I would be on ship and it would be sinking and I could not get up from the chair to save myself. The dreams involved a whole host of scenarios, but always the same result.

"I used to wake up and try to move my toes. I don't try now. My legs are as nothing, disconnected. From my feet, for example, I can feel nothing. I was warned not to cut my toenails myself. So I had to try, and I could cut them, feel nothing, and see the blood. It is a very strange experience. To realize that one can cut into one's flesh and see it bleed and yet feel nothing. To hurt yourself and not feel pain is amazing.

"Being with spinal cord injury is a different world with different rules; I just wish I knew what the rules are.

Early on, despite his feelings and explorations of his new body and new movements, he became impatient.

"Four to five weeks post injury I was awake and itching to mobilize. Early on progress is so slow; early on you are so slow. A million and one things come with spinal cord injury, like the muscle wasting. Within a week or so you become painfully thin, abnormally so. A mate was a warehouseman and now his arms are like sticks.

"Despite this, the relatives always say that their son, 'their boy' will get something back, even when told they may not, as though motivation can do it. It is being cruel to be kind to tell them this is not so. A young lad on the ward, just come in a week or so ago, age nineteen, was a guitarist. Music was his life. He had had two guitars with him since the injury: a good one and a knock about one. They told him that in all likelihood he would not play the guitar again. He was depressed and was crying for days. Then last week, Sister took one guitar from the bed into storage."

She had done it with the best of intentions, but the timing was brutal. Ian knew it was moving on too quickly. "It takes time to realize that this is not the end of the world."

Just as people need time to become accustomed to their new bodies, so it is clear that they need time to learn to move in the new ways necessary to care for themselves. An old cliché is that one's habits are for a lifetime. It is certainly the case that movement patterns, once developed, are there for many years. The way we walk, or tie our shoelaces, or our handwriting are all laid down and then used for years and years without thought. The trouble professionals can have in altering their golf swing testifies to how difficult such modifications of habits are.

People rehabilitating from spinal cord injury are faced with a number of movements and habits to learn for transfers, to eat, to write, to dress, and to look after their bladder and bowel. Just to balance in the chair or control their heads may require effort and concentration. These are also being done with weakened muscles or, in the case of balancing, with little or no muscle power below the neck. And all this has to happen when people are still vulnerable after their injury. Ian had puzzled over these problems for some time.

"Some things take a long time to learn. Say transfer from chair to bed; it used to take ages for me to use a board and move across. Now I do it without a board and almost without thinking. But it has taken nearly a year to get to that point. When your body settles down and the muscle groups settle, then things can improve a little."

For him one of the most difficult things was to learn to balance in a chair without postural muscles. This was made harder, in a way, because many people saw his hand function and presumed he was a paraplegic, with a level in the low cord, rather than a tetra. Balance and movement are not difficult simply because he is so weak. The lack of sensation in his body means that he has to look to see where he is. If the light is bad it is difficult for him to wheel around, because he has less idea where he is. To know quite whether he is upright and stable, he has to reference his position from a spot on the wall and work things out from that.

"When I am going up curbs or over streets, I have to stop people wheeling me, since if they do I cannot predict when I will move and so can become very unbalanced in relation to the world and my wheelchair, and I could fall out of it. Wheeling in the dark, I keep my elbows by my side so I can get a sense of where my upper body is in the chair. It is scary. You do not recognize it to start with. To understand it intellectually takes months."

All the time we were talking, Ian was gesturing not only with his arms and shoulders but also with his whole body in the chair. Almost unconsciously he was rocking it backward and forward as he spoke. Then he showed me how he did a wheelie, raising the front wheels of his chair and balancing backward a little, like motorcyclists do. What was impressive was that, as he did this, his eyes were absolutely still and focussed on an area on the wall in front of him. When rocking back he was absolutely dependent on referencing his position in the world from this area.

"When going up a curb I have to set my eyes on an object outside to know where I am in space. Going up a curb, you try to do it in one fluent move. You need the ability to do it and the confidence to do it without supervision. You have to move forward and once up drive on forward to prevent the head and neck going forward. It's like escalators in stores. I love doing it; people think you are mad. Up is easy; wheel on, grab handrails quick, if they move you let it drag you. Down, go backwards and grab the handrails quickly. It's a good stretch. Down is dodgy when the wheel hits the comb, since it can stop dead and you come out forwards, which is difficult. I do use the lifts, but I like people's reactions. Showing off."

Showing off. No one could begrudge him that. Even when talking to me he had moved from the despair of his early days to being ready to take on, explore, and almost play with his new body: He had recovered a joie de vivre.

A Voyage of Discovery

Not just wheelchair movement was difficult to master. Bowel and bladder took just as long.

"Things like intermittent catheterization—you can end up peeing on the bed and this can go on for months till you settle down to do it regularly and safely. When I first started doing it, I got a urinary tract infection, and my nurse Jacky gave me a real bollocking. I was trying the best I could, so I asked why since I washed my hands and did it the way I was shown. She said your technique is shit. That's the only way to make me listen."

He had been shown how to do it in a session and had followed instructions, but he was just not physically capable of doing all the new movements required in the right order and timing. For him to pass a catheter into his bladder while balanced on a chair, with weak hands and shoulders, a weak neck controlling his head, and with the problems of seeing what he was doing, were beyond his best efforts. But then slowly, after several months of doing it several times a day, he worked out a way.

"I now open the catheter, open a bit of sticky, split the packet, place it on loo, get a piece of tube, put that in my mouth while I get the catheter, shuffle forward on the chair, undo trousers and get everything out, connect, pass catheter and place over the loo. I do not know whether it [cognitive difficulty] is part of spinal cord injury, but it has taken me six months to do this simply. I would forget the order to do things. I would withdraw the catheter and urine would still bubble out. Now I rarely wash my hands. It is such a simple technique—and I do not have infections.

"Bowel care is the same and is a voyage of discovery. After two weeks, fourteen times, you would think you'd know what to do. But I would still have accidents and not know whether more would come down. Now, six months later, I am so comfortable with it. I know when I have finished and when I have not. I know what my body would do. You have to put a glove on and put your finger inside and move it round to stimulate evacuation, wait a little, and more will come down. Too much stimulation and too much will come out. I am constantly constipated, which is good, since it makes it easier. Despite it being explained and my doing it many times, it still took me months. All these things take time. The practical side is important.

"Imagine doing bowel care when your backside and two fingers are numb; it's a lottery. Doing bowel care I sit on a chair with a commode and I have to reach up between my legs, but then I lean forward, which is precarious, and I may fall forward, so I have to put my other hand on the sink or wall in front of me to stop me falling. It seems a long way forward, especially since if I go too far I have no postural muscles to stop me."

He also had to remember to put the brakes on first.[2]

"At the beginning I would not take a suppository and sit over the loo for hours and nothing. Then later that day I would have a power leak. Now I chuck the suppositories in and think nothing of it. But the chairs also pin your bum cheeks together, making it all so much more difficult. Then I keep dropping the suppositories, since they are so slippery. I just think it is funny.

"This is something that even the senior nurses don't appreciate, especially when they want you out of the loo. You can take an hour to do it and then clean up with a shower. Every now and then I have a problem and I ask for a check. Getting to know your own body or be in tune with it takes a long time. In normal life people do not listen to their body.

"Now I know when I need to self-catheterize my bladder. Normally I do it every four hours, but if I do not then I have learned what I need to know when the bladder is full. A slight feeling on the left hand side of low abdomen, just a mild tingling, is the sign. It is not a bloated bladder, but there is a definite sensation, nothing like I felt before.

"So I am thinking and playing with what I have left or have developed. I have tried limiting what I drink and leave it till 4 p.m., and at that time I will get the sensation and I will catheterize and get only 100 milliliters. So I am not sure what the sensation relies on. In a way it encapsulates spinal cord injury. So many things that most people do not have to think about or take for granted I have to."

A Turn-On

Much of this sounded pessimistic, yet it was clear from his way of saying it that Ian had a beautiful, dry, sense of humor.

"It's easy most of the time. I can get bitter, but only when the pain is so bad. Sometimes it gets bad and I am sardonic, often at my own expense. For instance, when the nurses are doing my bowel care, it is always the pretty ones. I find this so hard and so a bit of locker room or ward humor is the way through. It may say much about me, but the only way I can deal with it is through humor. It goes for the same on the ward. I would never dream of cracking the sort of jokes outside as we do here on the ward. When the pain is bad, the humor has more barbs and is often directed at me. Then we will have a night like tonight, when we go down town and have a few drinks, go to a club and flirt with some women, and life seems tolerable.

"Strangely enough, people have said that being in chair is a turn-on for some women, and that they come onto you, and it can be true."

I wondered if that was because men in wheelchairs are less threatening and less harmful. Yes, Ian explained, but—with a glint in his eye—this is not always the case, and when they found out it could be too late.

"Some guys in a wheelchair get drunk and so are the women, and things happen. I have had this experience since being injured. Viagra helps. The only thing you do not have is sensation . . . but there is more than one way to skin a cat. It puts you more attuned to the needs of the other, which is great. A young man's aim is to achieve orgasm. Later it is about the other person. One can ejaculate but, without wanting to sound too New Man about it, much of the pleasure has always been in your partner's pleasure, and that remains. The sense of closeness is still there and may be enhanced because of the spinal cord injury."

Though the sexual attraction was important for him and for his pride in himself, he hinted at something deeper.

"One of the saddest things for me is when it comes down to personal relationships. I have only just recently started discussing things with someone I really trust. When I meet someone, do they like me, because I am in a chair? They can't like me because I am in a chair. There are some things I can't do now and some I can, but it's still not the same. I have a constant nagging doubt. We go out to a pub and there is someone I am fond of and she is fond of me. I don't like to see the chair and feel so inadequate. She constantly tries to reassure me and say it does not matter. But I need to reassure myself, too.

"I think about the future: I picture some guy alone in a bungalow at the end of the road, behind lace curtains as the rain falls. That would be the end of my life, literally. One of my brothers took his own life some years ago. Men can't make a cry for help, they just do it. He did it in a way which was final, no going back. How he made that decision I will never know. I considered it. But my mother had three sons, and one died of cancer and another took his life. So I could not take my life while she was alive. I used to worry and wonder about the why and wherefore, but you get nowhere."

My Friend the Pain

Ian had talked for some time, over several occasions, but had not volunteered anything of his pain. I knew that he was on several drugs for pain and had tried many more, and that now he had an epidural pump, slowly passing drugs near the spinal cord itself. Was this because he could not describe the pain, or because he thought I would not be able to imagine it? In the end, I asked.

"My physical pain is in the hands and down the legs and in the feet. My hands hurt all over, related to the level of injury. The pain does not come on; it is there, the whole time, twenty-four hours per day every day, every day of the year. Most of the time I can override it, but I still know it is there. It is almost comfortable, almost my friend. I know it's there, it puts me in touch with my body. But when it's angry, it gets me so down. It can last twelve hours, or twenty-four or thirty-six. . . . I have just come through a bout last weekend and it was almost unbearable.

"It starts in the bottom and in the legs. It is hot, on the inside, like needles trying to get out. The feet feel as though someone has a bicycle pump on them, they feel massive as though they are about to explode, and then you look down on them and they are normal size, which is odd. They feel at least twice that size. That can drive you potty. Lying on the bed makes no difference. The worst is the undersides of my knees up to my buttocks, to my waist; buttocks and ankles drive me mad. With my buttocks, I am sure they are really hot and ulcerated, and yet they are not. At the same time, I get the feeling that my legs are ice cold, and I touch them and they are not, just numb and yet painful.

"Nothing makes it worse or better. I get into bed and try to lie on front or side. I am not sure it helps, but it makes me feel that I can do something about it. I have just got to get out of the chair. I go to the nurses' station and make them and me a cup of tea. As long as my hands are doing something, I feel a bit better. As soon as I sit there quietly again, the pain is there.

"There is no choice but to endure it. I have pain control with skin patches and tranidol and carbamazepine and the pump. But even with those, when it is bad it is bad. I cannot distract myself and watch TV. Since it happened, since I have been here, I have not been able to watch. I get up and go outside and have a cigarette, anything to distract myself. I have not had one comfortable night since it happened. I have not been nice and cozy. The pain is still there, and I cannot move, and in the middle of the night something will not feel right, and I just cannot feel right."

I asked if he ever woke up and forgot what happened—say, first thing in the morning.

"No, never, not even in dreams."

It must be extraordinary to have no feeling in the body and yet have the pain.

"I cannot do anything myself to get a connection. But despite that absence, I have to be aware of everything, since everything is dependent on me and my observation and thinking. For instance, if I reach out, my balance is so bad that I have to be aware I might fall. It is not natural, so I am aware the whole time. If I pinch my legs it is numb. The pain is the connection—my friend the pain."

It might have sounded as though Ian was so consumed by the pain and by the relatively new experience of living with spinal cord injury that he had little time for others, except the odd girlfriend. But this was not the case. He had put potted plants out in one of the hospital courtyards in the summer and watched the flowers grow and his strawberries ripen. The only thing he had grown previously, he told me, was cannabis. He kept this space, a small courtyard in the unit, *his* courtyard, clean and tidy and free of cigarette stubs. More, he had begun to care for others in the unit. He had built a cigarette holder based on a long wire and a clothes' peg for one man with an upper cervical injury so the man could hold his own cigarette. He had become an elder statesman and respected man around the wards.

Leaving

After a year in the hospital, Ian was concerned about what faced him outside. During his few trips outside, the physical challenges of access were all but impossible. I tried to reassure him that things had to get better.

"I don't think they will ever change enough. We are such a small section of society. When there are facilities you do feel better, as though you are a member of society again. I was around the front of the hospital recently, where they have just opened a new garden, and they asked me what I thought. I said I did not want to be negative, but it was terrible. The main entrance to the hospital is cobbled. No one with wheelchairs or prams can get over it. I was amazed. There are no curb cuts from the car park. Then the paving stones are staggered, so someone visually impaired would have big problems following them visually or even using a stick, since they are different levels.

"The five standing stones at the center of the new sculpture display need to be touched and yet no one in a wheelchair can get near them. I am absolutely staggered in terms of the absence of thought for disabled people in a hospital. It is elemental. They said that they had not thought it would be used by people in a chair."

The main event in people's lives recovering from spinal cord injury is their date of discharge. For the doctors, nurses, and occupational therapists there is much to consider, from whether the person is ready physically and emotionally, to the realization that too long inside can be counter-productive and lead to dependence. They also have to be aware that behind every person is another waiting for access to rehabilitation. Ian was given one discharge date, which passed by.

"They asked me to leave after six months or so. The doctor said, 'You can't stay here forever.' I felt desperate to leave, but not until I felt safe. A sister wanted me out since I was blocking a bed. I felt it personally. I could not go to a home. Their interest is in getting people through the unit and not with the end result. Once rehabilitated, they lose interest. Once out, I would have community liaison, theoretically, but I knew that I would be essentially on my own. No one has experience of spinal cord injury twice. They were trying to get me out too early. I am more than ready now."

This had been months ago, and he had little idea how the national health system worked and how he had to make it work for him. He needed to navigate his way through red tape to find a place to live and to obtain what grants there were. He hadn't a clue.

"When I came in, no one bothered to explain how the system works. I did not know what OTs do. Now I do; they get you to a point of living at home as independently as you can. Physiotherapists may do functional hand movement; they get your hands and muscles moving, but an OT will show you how to use the hands, getting joints moving and bulk up. With no feeling in the hands, a physiotherapist will not teach you how to use a cup, but an OT will, and will show you how to dress."

A physio once told me that they had a comparatively easy job, encouraging people to re-use what they can and to maximize what is left. They spend time with patients as they recover. Occupational therapists have to take this and apply it to the real world. They tread the much more demanding line between showing people the limits of what they will be able to do in a world which, for the most part, disregards disability, and encouraging, enabling, and empowering people to manage their environments to their best advantage.

Ian learned about the third mighty group, social workers, when he came closer to wanting to leave himself. In the hospital unit there were two excellent social workers, aware of the needs of people with spinal cord injury, but he soon came up against a housing department that was not.

"I need a double bed: not a want, a need. If I am to dress and transfer, I need a double bed. I can have a single in the hospital since I have back up if I fall. I need a double room, since I need a chair on one side and a commode or shower chair the other. My home housing department, and the social worker there, said that I was single and so had to have a single-room flat. I also need a chest of drawers and somewhere to put a spare wheelchair. So I have turned down one-bedroom flats. My OTs here realize the problem but cannot make the housing department understand it. As far as I can see, everyone leaving has this problem. I am lucky for a tetraplegic, since I have my hands. Without them I would need twenty-four hour care. A simple leather strap across the hands, and I can feed myself."

He has even been waterskiing with a group of paraplegics, struggling to keep up with them, rather than with his fellow tetraplegics.

"I am desperately trying to be independent. I don't want or need anyone in, unless I am ill. I have to make the housing department realize this. They suggested that if I fall out of a small bed, I could have a button to summon help. But a support network is no good. My Mum is old, and anyway it takes too long, and so I would have a pressure sore by the time anyone came to me. I asked them if they know what a spinal cord injury means, and they say yes, but clearly they do not.

"They give you a form, but initially you are not able to fill in a form. I was preoccupied with pain, with bladder, with my balance. For months I could not do forms. Being in a chair is the least of it. That would be acceptable if it wasn't for the bowel, bladder, sexual function, and pain and not being able to get access to things, and transport and difficulties in a pub if the bar is too high. Eventually there is the straw that breaks the camel's back (an unfortunate but apt metaphor). And it is not just the physical; the emotional aspect as well. The 'Does He Take Sugar?' syndrome constantly.[3]

"I am now having to chase the housing associations and negotiate with the housing department and their social workers, yet many still will not deal with me directly because I am a patient, yet the professionals here are not doing it. The top social worker I went to see was good at sympathizing. I was fuming at her, but within five minutes she had calmed me down: she had been on a course. I went to see a small flat. It was built in the 1960s for a single fit person, to minimum standards. How can a tetraplegic live in it?

"I have been ready to leave over the last two or three months. One day I had arranged to go to Exeter on the train, and was at the station and went dysreflexic: I had uncontrollable sweats above the injury and a burning in the bladder. My catheter was blocked, and so I tried a wash out in the station. If I had got on the train, my dysreflexia could have worsened, my blood pressure rocketed, and I might have had a stroke and been a basket case. I was desperate to go but could not and so I went back, and within ten minutes it was sorted out. I had realized it was bladder spasm, which I had never had before. I now know its symptoms and how it can be removed. I would have been stroked out. I felt unwell and thought it was my bladder, but once the catheter was unblocked I still had the burning, so I thought it was a bladder infection. But my nurse suggested it was a full bowel pressing on the bladder and irritating it, and hence the dysreflexia and sensation. How on earth are you supposed to know that, and then how can you tell a social worker unfamiliar with spinal cord injury why you did not show for the meeting?"

I was beginning to understand Ian's remark about the camel that broke the back. At first he was unready; now he was desperate to leave, but unable to because he could not convince the housing department of his reasonable needs. And he was having to do most of the work himself, with no knowledge of social services. He had had to learn as much about social services as he had about his body. He went on to tell me of another escapade he had recently enjoyed.

The Fertility Test

"Having the spinal injury has made me listen carefully to those helping me, and decide soon who I listen to and respect, and who I do not trust. I do not trust every nurse or doctor. It has been a complete education. I know more about me than many doctors and nurses, even within the unit. For example, I wanted a fertility test, since those with spinal injury have a low sperm count.

"We tried the more traditional ways of getting it without success. So they have this electric probe which is inserted up the anus and then turned on and it releases semen. I was told that I might have to 'milk the penis,' though I did not know what this meant. It was explained to me, quite funny really.

"When it came to it, the doctor asked if two female doctors could sit in. I said yes, since I wanted to help them with their education and partly because I was not really aware of what would happen. I lay down on my side, dropped my trousers, and the doctor slipped the probe into my backside and switched it on. I screamed straight away. He had told the doctors that you have to be very careful to avoid burning the inside of the anus. I screamed again and the doctor asked if I felt it. I explained, as calmly as I could, that yes I had, that I was C7 with some sensation, including some internal sensation.

"So he tried again and again. Each time was a form of torture. I have had electrical shocks before . . . but not there. Thank God the voltage was low. Anyway, I thought I would get an instant erection, but it was not the way.

"Then he said could you milk the penis, i.e., masturbate, or could we do it for you, which was acutely embarrassing. But also he had forgotten that I was left-handed and lying on my left side and arm. We had to move me round to lie on my right side to give me a free arm. We managed in the end and the sperm was OK; 10 percent Grade A, which is not bad.

"One female doctor was young and slim. I had to bite the bullet a bit. They seemed OK, but I felt they would tell their boyfriends. 'Milk the penis.' I was not aware I would have to masturbate in front of two women. And I was not aware that the penis would not be erect despite all this."

What was not clear at the time was why he wanted to go through all this, though to be considering his sperm count must have been a good sign. It was only later he told me he was having an affair with a barmaid in their local pub and that "only a few people knew." News like that would have spread like fire. Fortunately he had managed to be transferred from a four-bedded ward, with no privacy, to a single room in a halfway house. Even so, things had been dicey at times, not least because the barmaid was still living with her husband, though Ian assured me that the marriage was over. Just as well, I thought, as some husbands might not have seen the funny side of it.

He managed a chuckle. "Spinal cord injury. It's a funny old world." I said I was interested in what it is like to be someone else. He replied that having spinal cord injury is like being someone else. In a year he had learned a lot.

7 Exploration

Self and Others

The first thing that Ian considered was what he could not do, how he would no longer be independent, and how he would not have a family. All these, entirely appropriately, focussed on him and his loss. David's memories, admittedly from many years away, are of how he began to explore his new body and his new life as creatively as he could. Old hands in the treatment of spinal cord injured people say that the break may be the same, but the outcome for each person will differ according to his or her attitude.[1]

It is completely understandable that early on after a spinal cord injury the person concentrates on his or her own situation. For one thing, there are many new skills to learn. Living from a wheelchair, rather than being a relatively passive existence, needs a range of skills and judgements every bit as difficult as those we normally learn as children. We forget that we spent months and years learning to walk, climb, write, and even wipe our own bottoms. After spinal cord injury, many new skills are needed and have to be learned with the older, less flexible brains of adults. Ian spent months learning how to catheterize himself or manage his bowel. He was puzzled that these took as long as they did, but new movement skills are exceedingly difficult to learn as an adult. To have to do all these from a chair and with poor balance, no upper body movement and weakened arms, makes them immeasurably more difficult.

Eventually, people begin to look around. But this too can be difficult. Robert Murphy described how his paralysis had altered his self-other balance profoundly. He felt a desire to shrink from society and fall back into himself.

With their adult lives before them, neither Ian nor David felt quite such a pull. But they did go through phases of introspection and doubt. David, fresh from university, got on with life most successfully for a decade before his second major physical illness precipitated a period of soul searching. Ian, in contrast, spent months in the hospital looking inward, before beginning to look around and take an interest in others. In this he is quite similar to a man that Nigel North, a clinical psychologist, told me about.

"This man, a plumber, was very good at his job, and prided himself on his accuracy and speed. He was focussed on being strong, physical, agile, and above all quick. His whole view of the world was this. He had been paralyzed from the neck down for ten months, and for the first six could not talk about how it felt nor access what he was like. He would just say it is awful, more bluntly than that. 'I am not going to be anyone; I am useless, on the scrap heap.'

"Very gradually he began to talk about his feelings of being in the spinal unit, about looking at others and feeling the tragedy of other people and wanting to talk to them about how they felt. Almost imperceptibly he developed a language of emotion and care. It sounds as though I am saying he did not care before, when he did, but his vision was focussed on work, and on him, and now it has changed and is now about talking with people and supporting them. And talking to them about things he still has, like his feelings of sadness or euphoria. He is trying to understand his purpose in life now. What will it be for now that he has left his plumbers' world behind? He has a new language."

For Ian too the injury and change in circumstances had required him to explore other aspects of himself, and arguably may have made him more social. David had bounced back from his injury brilliantly and had enjoyed the next decade almost by ignoring his spinal cord injury as best he could. This had been very successful, and he looks back on those years with great affection. Then, however, the combination of several severe illnesses and surgical operations brought him to a very low state, made so much worse by the erroneous information about his likely lifespan. Under the circumstances, few people would find the resources to keep going. Yet there may have been other factors involved.

After ten years, he felt he had created very little. He had no relationship, no permanent place to live, and had largely lived his life for him. In the sessions with the psychologist, he explored ways to change. He decided not only to move out from his parents' house, but also to become active in the field of disability. He was no longer denying his body, but beginning to explore it and explore how he could help others. He wrote a manual of how to live with spinal cord injury, and he became an advocate. In this he is keen not to be portrayed as a saint, or as someone whose own worth comes from helping others. After all, he has enjoyed himself abroad and done lots of other things for himself alone. But part of his return to a social existence has been to find a world in which he has value, not just in his immediate circle, but also in much wider areas of health provision and resources.[2] He has not turned his back on his old world and his old friends—in fact, his warmth and sociability has made him a focal point for old university friends—but his new world, embracing his impairment, has allowed him to see his abilities and worth.

Nothing So Isolating

The most obvious aspects of spinal cord injury, mobility, and perhaps loss of sensation, may be less important than problems with continence and pain. Chronic pain, which is usually beyond help from medications, is a completely different experience from acute pains some of us may have had. Chronic pain can ruin a life and make people question their very existence.[3]

People with spinal cord injuries may experience an almost bewildering number of pains. Some come on at the time of the injury, due to co-incident injuries elsewhere. This acute pain can usually be treated, but damage to the spinal roots and nerves associated with the injury can lead to pain at and around the level of injury that may continue for years. This "root pain" is much more difficult to treat.

Later, other pains may also emerge. Muscle spasms can be acutely painful and, being temporary bursts, are difficult to predict or treat.

Visceral pain within the abdomen may sometimes reflect renal or bladder problems. Another pain, which Colin experienced so badly, is due to acute high blood pressure, causing severe headache and rendering the patient at risk of a stroke.

People with spinal injury spend their lives transferring between car and chair, bed and shower. Each transfer requires them to hump their full weight with their shoulders. It is therefore not surprising that they can develop severe joint problems. Arthritis, which might be tolerable in a mobile person, becomes a big problem in someone who has to transfer using his or her shoulders.

Last, and possibly the cruellest pain of all, is deafferentation pain, felt below the level of the injury in an area the person cannot feel or move. This develops weeks to months after the initial spinal cord injury and may be the response of the spinal cord and brain to the absence of a sensory input. Though originating within the central nervous system, it is felt in the legs, feet, buttocks, anywhere below the injury.

There have been many studies of the prevalence and severity of pain in spinal cord injury. Most suggest that 60–70 percent of people with spinal cord injury have pain, and that it is considered severe in 20–30 percent.[4,5] Pain is difficult to quantify, and so some studies have sought to see its effects on individuals.[6,7] In a large postal survey of 885 people, Rose et al. found that 43 percent had constant pain.[6] Pain rather than immobility prevented work in 98, stopped social activities in 118, and interfered with sleep in 325.

It is scarcely surprising that such chronic pain has an effect on quality of life, though for some years the medical professional, unable to treat it, downplayed its significance. When Rose's paper was submitted to a spinal cord journal in 1987, it was rejected because patients could not be expected to be able to analyze their own pain objectively or scientifically. Fortunately, times have changed, and pain treatment is now much more of a focus.[8]

Moderate pain, felt in the unsentient and unmoving part of the body, may give some feeling of connectedness. But it is clear also that severe pain is a major problem in many with spinal cord injury and can alter the fragile balance between enjoying and enduring life. Yet several people I spoke with did not mention their pain unless I asked. It was just something they kept to themselves, knowing there was no good treatment and not wanting to focus on it. One man only mentioned his pain a year or so after we met. It was not bad, a 2 or 3 on a scale of 10 most of the time, he said, but still tiring. At work he would long for lunch or for 5 p.m. just so that he could relax from the mental effort of managing pain and work at the same time.

By its very nature, pain is a private experience, without external referent and without a clear, shared vocabulary, despite many useful word lists.[9] That is why, however much one tries to take in figures and graphs and words of pain, it is the personal, lived experience of it that is most compelling. At a meeting on pain in spinal cord injury, a distinguished lady sat in her wheelchair and carefully and slowly described her own pain. It was as though "someone has wrapped my legs in barbed wire and then passed an electric shock through them." She added that paralysis does not stop life, but pain may.

No wonder Murphy wrote that "Nothing is quite so isolating as the knowledge that when one hurts, nobody else feels the pain."[10] To have such pain when living in a chair, with less opportunity for distraction, must make it even more difficult. All the more amazing how Ian has picked up his life despite having to live with such severe pain.

It's Not the Respirator, It's the Money

David had gone ten years with his spinal cord injury without thoughts of suicide. When he did consider it, he judged his life unworthy and rationalized this in terms of his spinal cord injury. In retrospect, it is clear that this was triggered by his illnesses and by his erroneous thought that his lifespan was nearly run.

The rate of suicide among those with spinal cord injury is roughly five times that of the general matched population, with most of these in the first five years after the injury.[11] Many may consider suicide soon after their injury, before they have explored and adapted to their new lives, or a little later, when setbacks disturb the delicate balance of costs and benefits of living. Later still, people discover a richness and enjoyment in life, with different interests and pleasures.

I discussed suicide with a group of physiotherapists. They thought it was not necessarily a terrible thing; patients had to decide for themselves. One described a fit man who had worked for the FBI. After his spinal injury, he did all his rehab and built up arm movements and muscle bulk, just so that he was capable of turning a gun on himself.

Another young man had found that he would be ventilator dependent. He was diabetic and asked not to take his insulin. His doctors respected his wishes after several psychiatrists agreed that he was mentally competent.

A recent very high profile case in the United Kingdom was that of Miss B. She had had a brain hemorrhage a year or so before and was completely paralyzed and needed ventilation. She had asked for the ventilator to be turned off, but her medical team, who had known her for several months, refused, believing she might change her mind. But she had had enough. A judge agreed with her. She was moved to another hospital and the vent stopped, with the appropriate drugs to prevent her from more suffering. Her doctors had argued that with further time and rehabilitation and placement in her own home, with support, she might have decided life was worthwhile. The figures suggest that they might have had a point, though of course applying general figures to individual situations can never be precise.

Paul Kennedy analyzed the people who had committed or attempted suicide from Stoke Mandeville from 1951–1992.[12] He found 134 cases, with an equal spread between men and women. Half were single, a third had children, and perhaps surprisingly, 42 percent were employed. Most of these attempted to end their life by falling. He also found a high prevalence of schizophrenia and depression. His analysis was complicated by the fact that some tetraplegics may have caused their injury by falling from windows in an earlier suicide bid.

Because of the reduced number of ways unassisted suicide can be attempted with tetraplegia, there have been a number of high profile cases, especially in the United States, in which tetraplegics have asked for help. Jenny Morris quotes the case of a historian and disabled woman, Elizabeth Bouvia.[13] She was a "twenty-six-year-old woman, attractive and educated." She checked herself into a hospital psychiatric unit and announced her wish to commit suicide. She reported that she had had two years of devastating emotional crises: the death of a brother, serious financial distress, withdrawal from graduate school because of discrimination, pregnancy and miscarriage, and, most recently, the breakup of her marriage. She said that the main reason for wanting to die was her physical disability. Three psychiatric professionals concluded that she was mentally competent and that her decision for death was reasonable. Ignoring her emotional problems, they based their judgement on one fact alone—her physical handicap.

Jenny Morris mentions others with spinal injury who were adjudged mentally competent to end their own lives, including the infamous McAfee case. He was tetraplegic, ventilator dependent, and claimed that he had enough. The lawyers agreed, again based on his disability. It turned out that he had severe financial problems and concerns over where and how he would live. As the case unravelled, he announced that his problem was "not the respirator. It's the money."

One must be careful not to assume that the cord injury is the sole cause for the petition for suicide, when other life events might be the real reason. One problem, from the outside, is that we should never try to think what we would think in that position, from our own perspective, but try to see the situation from the position of the person in it. The problem may sometimes be one of empathy.[14,15,16] Morris discusses these issues from the perspective of the "disabled movement": "We [the disabled] are sometimes ourselves guilty of undermining the lives of [other] disabled people. Those of us who walk with crutches often think to have to use a wheelchair would mean life was not worth living, and those who do use a wheelchair but have use of our arms and hands think that to be completely paralyzed would be sufficient reason to commit suicide. . . . We are undermining the lives of those who are already more disabled than ourselves."

She considers that we need to support the right of disabled to take their life if they want to, but be cognizant of the fact that it might not simply be the physical disability that was determining and defining their wants. Morris suggests that many such cases are often couched in terms of civil rights, with lawyers being concerned to accede to and "win" the disabled the legal right to die. In her view however, "Given the level of prejudice against disabled people, we cannot realistically expect non-disabled journalists or the medical profession, or the legal profession, to mount a challenge to the assumption that a physical disability means a life not worth living. We [disabled people] have to challenge it ourselves."

One can, of course, agree with the sentiments expressed, though this particular battle may have been won within spinal cord injury services—I did not meet anyone who would disagree with Morris. We cannot deny people the chance to end their lives if that is their choice and if other complicating factors have been excluded (accepting that this has to be done with great thoroughness). According to Nigel North, the clinical psychologist, "Some have decided that their life is not worth living. After I have tried to get them to look differently or explore different things or feel differently, then if someone is really saying that my life is not worth it, there are hoops to jump through with independent psychiatrists. I have helped them ease the path. People make these decisions with a large amount of thought. I don't take it lightly, but if after six months to a year they are still firm, then . . ."

His voice tailed off and then he began once more, this time more positively. "I have often used someone with a similar injury who has managed to create a life for themselves. Some I know have been very depressed but, gradually, have found a quality of life they like. One of the things I know is that because I do not have a spinal cord injury, whatever I say, I cannot know what it is like to have one. I would never presume to know what it is like. But someone who has an injury and been despairing and then managed to create a life is a very powerful advocate for life."

Enjoying

"Neurology's favourite word is 'deficit,' denoting an impairment or incapacity . . . loss of speech, loss of vision, loss of dexterity and a myriad other lacks and losses."[17] There can be few losses so complete as those in spinal cord injury, with its loss of movement, of sensation, of orgasm, and of continence. Loss, however, is only one side of the impairment. There are a huge number of medical issues consequent on the injury, including pressure sores, infections, and especially chronic pain.

Thus far we have focussed on deficits and problems, not only to show the problems but also to give measure to the achievements of those who put their lives back together. And yet, despite all these problems, Ian and David, after a time of reflection, began to explore new ways of living in a myriad of creative ways. Within a year or so, Ian was riding the escalators in his chair for fun, able to joke about his first attempts at catheterization and, of course, confident enough for a relationship. If slower, then

David had, after a long period of self-examination, reestablished his life and doubted whether he would really want to be restored. Despite everything, they were relishing life. In this they are not unusual, for most people with spinal injury discover and create enrichment and enjoyment.

Stensman asked people with spinal cord injury how they viewed and enjoyed their lives once they have been discharged from their hospitals and rehab clinics.[18,19] The mean value of self-reported quality of life was 8.0, which differed only slightly from controls' 8.3. Functions lacked by the disabled persons were rated as less important, and they took pleasure from different things, with more time for cultural and social activities. He interviewed a group of seventeen people with complete traumatic spinal cord injury on six separate occasions, from six months to five and a half years after their injury, a total of 102 interviews. Four patterns of response were seen, with five subjects coping very well, with an almost unchanged assessed quality of life after the injury; six were coping well after an initially low period. It may take several years to adjust to spinal cord injury. A further two subjects reported that their qualities of life were unstable, whereas four reported a low quality without improvement. Those with low ratings had severe pain, were older at the time of trauma, and felt blameless for the accident.[20] Another survey also found quality of life among people with spinal cord injury good, with 93 percent glad to be alive and only 10 percent judging their lives to be poor or very poor.[21]

After the initial trauma and the months of rehab, it may take a few years to sort out home and life, but after these adjustments a good quality of life is possible and indeed probable.[22] In one study of those with spinal cord injury,[23] quality of life was found to be related to a list of nine variables: physical function and well-being, independence, accessibility, spontaneity, emotional well-being, stigma, relationships, social function, and occupation and finances—just like the rest of us.

Underlying some of the discussions of spinal cord injury has been the relationship between our body and our perceived self, and how this may be altered in tetraplegia. As we have seen, the body is not absent from attention in tetraplegics and, though lacking movement and sensation, may require more attention toward its biological needs for pressure care and urination.

Historically, once movement was lost it could not be reclaimed. But now, for the first time, there have been successful attempts to restore movement to paralyzed parts. In the next section, we meet two women who have been involved in trials to recover movement, either to regain use of a hand in tetraplegia or to recover standing in the case of paraplegia. These experiments not only allow practical advantages to the subjects but also allow some reflection on the relationships between our sense of ownership of our bodies and our sense of owning movement. If we see our leg moving under computer control, do we feel alienated from it or feel a reclaimed sense of embodiment within a part of ourselves reawakened from paralysis?

In the next chapter, Julie Hill describes how she managed to stand as a complete paraplegic using her own legs, and in the chapter following, Deborah Graham discusses her feelings at having function in her right hand after several years of paralysis.

IV

Experimenting

8 Because I Can

Though she may not like it, Julie Hill is one of the most famous spinal cord injured people in the United Kingdom. She was the first person to have an elaborate series of electrodes implanted to stimulate the nerve roots as they leave the spine, below the level of her injury, allowing her movement in her previously paralyzed legs. But there is much more to Julie than being a guinea pig, and in her autobiography[1] it is not until page 213—out of 289—that she reaches the operation that led to her fame. Though her publishers insisted in their blurb on writing about "how science helped turn tragedy to triumph," and of her "mak[ing] medical history," Julie actually tells her personal story on living with spinal injury candidly and with deceptive simplicity.

I've Always Wanted to Be in a Helicopter

A tire burst as she accelerated to overtake a car. She was flung from her car, flew over a bank, and landed in a field. One of her first memories, apart from of the pain in her back, was that she could not feel her legs. When twenty minutes or so later the emergency services arrived, she was distressed, thinking her legs were sticking up in front of her, revealing more than she wanted.[2] "Please put my legs down, they're in the air." After a night at the local hospital, she was airlifted to the Spinal Centre at Salisbury. She told her Dad, "I've always wanted to be in a helicopter." Somewhere she heard her mother break down again.

Later, after a stabilization operation on her spine and days of searing back pain only intermittently relieved by opiates, she understood what had happened. Her spinal cord was severed in the mid-thoracic level (T9). Not bruised, not stretched, but severed, so there was no equivocation about prognosis. With a complete paralysis and loss of sensation from the waist, she knew she would never walk again.

I had completely ruined my life. . . . I was going to be a burden to everyone. . . . Kevin would probably leave me—or, if he stayed, it would only be out of some noble sense of obligation. The children would grow up with the social impediment of a wheel chair bound mother. I was a useless cripple. Disabled. Damaged goods. (p. 34)[3]

Her nurse tried to point out some positive aspects, and the fact that she was lucky in being affected from the waist down only—many in her ward were tetraplegic. Julie tried desperately to see it like that, but for some time she was consumed with anger and self-pity, particularly about her prospects for sex. Her anxiety was defused a little by a New Zealand nurse whose accent made it sound as though they were discussing "oral six."

Then her leg swelled due to a blood clot. Apart from anything else—it was, after all, life threatening—this new obsession with her legs, she wrote, did nothing to help her come to terms with the loss of their use.

I would sit staring at them, willing them to work, the sweat beading on my forehead with effort and concentration. Perhaps through sheer will and bloody-minded determination I could make them move again. It was several days before I realised it was pointless. I had irreversibly severed the connection between my thought processes and the muscles. (p. 120)

Her bladder problems and urinary incontinence were more distressing. She describes the arrival of the first visitors; an ordeal, until they saw that she was not *"a dribbling, gibbering wreck who smelt of stale urine. . . . Once they saw my smiling face, the relief on their own was evident, and after that we just did our best to carry on as usual."* (p. 94)

"As usual," though, was relative. The early morning round for staff to evacuate bowels manually was one of the lowest of points, as was her first menstrual period. Then came her first wheelchair. The staff were pleased, because it allowed her an escape from bed. Julie, in contrast, was appalled; the chair would define her from now on.

When you are sick, you are in bed in hospital. When you are better, you get up and go home. . . . This was it; my prison for the rest of my life. . . . I loathed the chair. . . . Catching a glimpse of myself in a full-length mirror . . . the broken body, slumped in the ugly apparatus which was to be my outer skin for the rest of my life. . . . My self esteem hit rock bottom. (pp. 113–114)

Julie describes her family seeing her in the chair, with her husband stony faced and fearful and her mother bursting into tears. But then came the reaction of her two boys, aged four and six, something Julie was dreading most. They just grinned from ear to ear and demanded a ride around the ward. The chair was just another way of getting their Mom around.

There followed several months of learning to be a paraplegic, with new routines and safety measures to learn.

A Different Person?

Going home proved to be another ordeal, but one away from the security of her ward. She felt she made the house untidy with her various medical appliances. She came in with mud on her wheels. Her bladder was still misbehaving and, to establish continence, she needed several operations. For her first year she was in the hospital as much as at home, and home became increasingly foreign. She describes months of trying to re-establish herself as mother and wife when she felt particularly vulnerable and like a stranger.

If home was a trial, then the "real world" was worse. She would go shopping with her mother, hand over money, and watch as the cashier handed change back to her Mom. People would ignore her in conversation at school gates, though she soon found how to stop it through humor and frankness. She told one mother, "I can see right up your nose." Fussing husbands, fussing parents, concerned friends also had to be put at ease. She had to introduce her new friends, in wheelchairs, very carefully at home to Kevin. Their presence served to accentuate the distance between him and Julie.

In her book, Julie does not avoid these problems. Many—if not most of them—were from other people rather than from the spinal cord injury. *"I was still the same person inside, I still thought the same and felt the same. . . . But everyone seemed to regard me as a different person.*

I was an invalid, a stranger. It was as if my accident had erased their memories of me." (p. 143)

At home and away from the unit, it is clear just how Julie struggled. Her recovery, she thinks, began with a remarkable weekend away with a charity, Back Up, providing sport for people with spinal injuries. They do not provide archery and basketball; her first trip was a four-day waterskiing weekend, and soon after she was abseiling and sailing.

Once you've got up on a sitz ski (an elongated knee board) and gone once round a lake . . . all your preconceived ideas of what disability is about go flying. I was terrified and then totally exhilarated . . . it changed my attitude to my disability almost overnight. (p. 154)

Back home she began to take more care of herself, to care for herself once more. How she looked, what she wore, began to matter.

The Reciprocal Gait Orthosis

Two years after her injury, Julie saw an article in a paper about a young policeman, Police Constable Olds, who had become paraplegic during a raid when a bullet went through his spine. He had vowed to walk again, and newspapers eagerly bankrolled his attempts, feeding off his publicity. For this macho young man, walking was all. When all the options failed, he committed suicide.

This article discussed a new technique he had tried, the reciprocal gait orthosis, or RGO. It was a sort of giant clothes peg. The patient is placed in two leg braces with a close fitting body brace that allows a scissoring, puppetlike "walk" as one leg is swung forward with the body and arms. It is tight, very difficult to get into and out of, and clumsy. But it does allow paraplegics to "stand," or at least be upright and swing along a little.

The staff at Salisbury arranged for Julie to have one. But she needed help in and out of it, and it was hot, uncomfortable, and, rather than allowing her less visibility, was profoundly unflattering and attracted attention. It was easier and more socially acceptable to get around in a chair. After a few months of effort, she abandoned the RGO. However, it had given her a taste for experimentation—and for standing.

Help Wanted

A little while later, in 1993, Julie was reading a magazine for the spinally injured and saw a call for volunteers for a new form of stimulation, functional electrical stimulation (FES) of the spinal roots. Previous FES had involved electrodes attached to the muscles or nerves in the leg. This had always proved difficult; few nerves and muscles were accessible, and the electrodes were difficult to place and keep in the right place. Implanting electrodes next to the nerve roots, as they came out from the spinal cord deep within the body, promised better and more stable stimulation and less hassle, at least after the operations. The scientific team thought this new system, lumbosacral anterior root stimulator implant (LARSI), might allow standing.

But more, Julie saw immediately, the absence of wires would make any FES movement seem more natural to her than a giant clothes peg or a battery of wires.

"I had tried callipers [crutches], fine but bloody hard work. They were a means to an end but mechanical and cumbersome. The FES system looked a good alternative. It would use my muscles again, part of me rather than a framework. To have that implanted with no wires, all within, made it more me. Just as I had a bladder operation to get rid of leg bags, if it's more me in control then that is good for me mentally."

She applied and was accepted onto the program as one of a group of possible candidates for the first trial. Though eight or so were planned, there was only money initially for one, so there was a competition to be first. She began a long series of assessments and exercises. Her bones were measured for density, to make sure they could stand her weight after years without use. Her spine was X-rayed to make sure there was room to operate, and her skin assessed for resistance to pressure sores. For nine months, up to three hours a day, she used external FES to build up her wasted muscles. She was on a mission and determined to be first. Eventually, with the external FES and built-up muscles, under supervision, she could stand. When she did it in front of her kids, she was amazed how small they looked from high up. She graduated to standing for up to ten minutes at a time, though beyond that was difficult because the muscles became fatigued and cramped.[4]

In the end, the team had to decide which of two patients was to be the first. The decision was close, but it went to Julie.

The research team were very experienced and ingenious. They had previously developed a variety of neural prostheses, including early cochlear implants and a visual implant to try to stimulate the visual cortex in the brain directly to imitate vision. They had also made an implanted FES system for paraplegics, with electrodes stimulating various peripheral nerves, but breakages and infection had dogged the project. They had invented a device for allowing semen collection in men with spinal cord injury, allowing them a chance of fatherhood. But probably their most famous invention was a sacral root stimulation system, enabling urinary continence and voiding to command that has transformed the lives of hundreds with spinal injury.

The surgeons and physiotherapists were in Salisbury, but the engineers remained in the background in London. Their design was for a set of twelve electrodes fitted around the nerve roots, and then taken under the skin to the receiver placed over the ribs. Over this, on the skin, would be placed a programable transmitter. To implant this, the local surgeon, Tony Tromans, was spending his spare time practicing in the hospital mortuary.

By the time Julie had been selected, the idea that a paraplegic would be made to stand without external wires or braces had become news. A TV crew had picked up on it even before the decision about who the first patient should be. They complicated the choice between the final two by suggesting that Julie might be the more photogenic. This did not sway the team—almost the reverse, in fact.

The night before the operation, in December 1994, Julie met the main boffins for the first time as Nick Donaldson and David Rushton came down from London. They wanted to give Julie one last chance to reconsider. With the unit, the scientists, and the TV crew, as well as her family and friends all caught up in the project, they were very aware that Julie might have found it difficult to back out. She had no such thoughts.

The operation took nine hours, as Tony identified each nerve root and then carefully, guided by a subtle difference in color, separated the unneeded sensory fibers from the crucial motor, or movement, ones. Working in a small field of two centimeters or so, he had to find each of twenty nerves and then place them singly on a small electrode to allow the engineers to see which muscle group twitched when they were stimulated. In this way, they slowly and carefully identified each root and then attached a small permanent electrode to it, sealed the whole area, and led the electrodes to the receiver.

Turning On

It took Julie several days to recover from such a long operation. Then · came the big moment. The doctors, nurses, boffins, TV crew, and family crowded into a room. Slowly, they stimulated an electrode through the transmitter and watched. Despite their operative measurements, they were not entirely sure which muscle group would move from a given electrode. Indeed, initially, they were not sure which leg it would be. *"I have never felt so many eyes boring into me. All attention was on my legs and I was willing them to move as hard as anyone."* (p. 228)

The first trial was of the knee extensor, quadriceps.

Everyone continued to stare as the various muscles in my thigh (including quadriceps) contracted and lifted my leg an inch.
"Tell us if that's at all uncomfortable, won't you?"
"No," I said, still beaming, "That's fine, Wow!"
This was it, this was what we had all been working towards and it felt absolutely brilliant. There were no wires, no visible electrodes, nothing, just me and my skin and some pretty complicated and expensive gadgetry a few feet way. OK, the electrical input was coming from outside, but it was my nerves working my muscles lifting my leg for the first time in four years. Mine, and without any encumbrances. I was back in control and it felt wonderful. I caught my father's eye and he winked at me. It was all I could do to stop the tears from spilling.
"You're enjoying this, aren't you, Julie?"
"Thoroughly," I exclaimed, understating the case wildly.
We tried again and again. . . . At one point my leg was raising itself off the bed and bending rhythmically in a sort of can-can. It was absolutely brilliant, although by the time the switch on test had been completed an hour later, I was physically shattered, I was still almost beside myself with delight. (pp. 229–230)

She had spent nearly a year making her muscles strong again. Her paralyzed body had been transformed through external FES. This had preoccupied her day after day, and now her body was moving without external stimulation. She willed the movement, and here before her eyes success was visible. *"My* nerves, *my* leg, *Mine."* All twelve electrodes worked, and there had been no damage to the nerves from the operation. Everyone was on a high.

Next came long series of experiments trying to find the best combinations of stimuli to produce movement. When we stand normally there are complex patterns of activation of muscles across pelvis, hip, knee, and ankle joints. Though people had recorded muscle activity during standing before, no one had attempted to reproduce it from stimulation and no one knew which combinations, strengths, and timings to use. The sessions were long and boring for Julie. Tiring too, for her muscles were being stimulated the entire time. Even though she was not putting her own intellectual effort into it, she was doing the physical work; she was out of breath at times, and frequently covered in sweat.

By February, they were ready for the first stand between parallel bars. The team and the TV crew gathered again, as Tim, the electronics engineer, turned on the channels. Slowly Julie rose. But her hips were kinked to one side and she was very unstable. Julie could hardly balance, let alone stand. It was worse than the external FES and a real anticlimax, as big a low as the first turn-on had been a triumph. They tried desperately, burdened by the extra pressure of a TV crew keen for a happy ending.

There followed long series of experiments to sort out the best combinations of muscle stimuli to allow Julie to stand. But the problem was evident with the first turn-on; a given nerve root supplied muscles with various actions, so that stimulation led to knee straightening and also to hip flexion, leading to her body jackknifing. They had to see if they could give some power to one set of muscles without leading to other muscles negating the effect.[5] These long sessions, over months, were especially draining for Julie. *"Each session lasted from 10 a.m. till 4 p.m. At times I felt like a pair of legs and nothing more. . . . I called the depression I sank into at this stage 'guinea pigiitis'."* (p. 241)

The Multi-moment Chair

Her hopes, once huge, drained slowly from her. The team found it difficult to know the force each muscle and each stimulation produced. How could one measure force in so many muscles acting at several joints? They arranged a crude system involving bathroom scales placed under the moving leg, but to understand the forces from stimulation they had to measure the torque across each joint. Nick Donaldson had anticipated this and developed a device called a multi-moment chair. This would allow them to computerize the movements, forces, and torques following stimulation and, they hoped, allow a refinement of Julie's stimulation parameters. A slight problem was that Julie was more moveable than the chair; so once or twice a month she made the two-hundred-mile round trip to North London.

The chair was *"Ten feet long by three feet wide, made of wood and metal and weighing a quarter of a ton. I came to hate it. Like a whole-body straightjacket, I was strapped tightly into it . . . my feet were strapped into in, my knees were clamped and restrained. . . . There would follow hours upon hour of tests while I lay back watching them or reading a book. The only respites were for lunch, tea or coffee. . . . Apart from the odd amusing moment it was totally boring, from ten in the morning to six at night."* (pp. 242–243)

The program was more complicated and more tiring than she ever imagined. Each time it was like a full body workout for Julie, because the leg muscles were being activated intermittently for up to six hours. She was so tired that she often could not drive home; sometimes she fell asleep during the tests.[6]

The team was discovering fascinating details, but she began to hate the machines. It all seemed so far from her needs of standing and using the LARSI system in her daily life at home.

While scientific careers were being forged, I felt more and more like a tooth in a cog in a wheel. . . . All I wanted was some sort of tangible result. . . . There were times when I felt quite trapped by the situation I had put myself into. . . . I could not leave, I didn't want to most of the time, but there were times when it really got to me. Session after session, I stood and sat, stood and sat, stood and sat, sweat pouring off me with the exertion, as they measured and graded. . . . I don't think I had ever realised how physically and emotionally exhausting the whole process would be. (pp. 246–247)

There were, however, some parts that continued to interest Julie. They were all surprised that she could feel stimulation from an area considered insentient since the injury. *"When I am being electronically stimulated, I can somehow tell what position my legs are in, even though I still have no feeling in them. But if the current is off, and I close my eyes, and my legs are manually manipulated, I have no idea whether they are straight or bent."* (p. 247)

Overall though, her patience and her hopes were running low. At one stage, frustrated by the absence of progress, she gave the team an ultimatum; she wanted something for herself or she would quit. They switched their programs and aimed for some short steps rather than standing. With much effort, this was barely achieved. She was the first person with paraplegia to stand without any external stabilization or wires, and the TV program ended with her at a bar of a pub ordering a drink. But she knew how much effort it was, and how unstable she was.

To avoid activating unwanted muscles during stimulation they tried injecting those muscles with anaesthetic, and then with a temporary paralyzing agent, botulinum toxin. Neither were very successful, because it was not just a single muscle that was the problem but several and, in any case, a muscle that might not be needed for one movement might be needed for another. They were running into the sand.

Media Star

Paradoxically, just as the project was stalling, the TV film of the operation and her progress came out. Suddenly she was a media star. Julie was featured in countless newspaper articles and TV shows, and was given an award at the 1996 European Women of Achievement awards. This interest did make the somewhat disheartened team realize just what they had achieved, something that was sorely needed. But equally, the coverage in the papers and on TV was sensationalist, with headlines such as "Walking Miracle."

In giving interviews, Julie was always very careful. Interviewers imposed their ideas on her: that she wanted to walk to appear normal and no longer be disabled. She would correct them as best she could, saying that the system allowed standing and possibly some steps but not walking. But usually they did not listen.

"The media and especially the tabloids were horrendous. They expected me to walk again, and though I took some steps, it was never going to replace the chair. They wanted a story. I was headline news and I was saying, 'No, no.' I would always say this will not replace the wheelchair, but it has given me a choice. I would be like a parrot saying it. 'If I don't stand up then I won't, but I could if I wanted; it is my choice.'

"Walking is not the be all and end all. It is too bloody hard and difficult, and what is the point? I am very able in my chair. LARSI has given me the opportunity to stand if I want to—not very well and not as it should be. That is where we might have failed, but the keeping fit all makes me feel good about myself."

Where the media could have debated mobility in people with neurological impairments, they focussed only on walking and how Julie might have escaped being disabled and be returned to the fold of the normal. Even better for the story, there was a good team of boffins and doctors in the background to explain and fulfill their role.

Tricycle Time

The frenetic period of research and practice could not be sustained. Julie's life continued and needed some independence from the LARSI. Then, one day, seeing the boys off on their bikes with Kevin, she suddenly thought that she might cycle with the LARSI system. She would not have to balance or stand, her weight would be supported, and the movement itself ought to be easier, with no problems of hip stability. She immediately phoned the team. They were equally enthusiastic.

They tried her on a simple bicycle wheel and found that controlling leg circling with FES was "relatively" simple. Over the next few months, the project was rejuvenated as they adapted a tricycle. One of the problems with FES is that though the implant controlled muscle activation, it had no feedback from the legs or from the relation between legs and the ground. On a bike, feedback could be provided from the position of the pedals, a huge advantage in movement design and control. They rapidly designed a system allowing measurement of pedal rotation and of the force applied to each pedal. This was fed back to the computer, determining the correct activation of muscles.

Soon Julie had a portable system allowing her to cycle short distances. Her first outdoor ride was in a nearby forest, with her two boys beside her. To feel the sun on her face and wind in her hair as she went down a track with the boys would have been unimaginable a year before. Now it was just beautiful. It was also a richly deserved triumph for the team looking on. They had worked so hard for so many years. Here, at last, was something that might be used out of the lab.

Because I Can

Julie and the team's commitment to the whole project was huge. At one time there were six full-time researchers plus many other people giving parts of their time. There were major grants from the United Kingdom's two main physiological and medical research charities. For Julie, "I have had a lot of people say why bother? The answer is always because I can."

But there is more. Paraplegics often like muscle spasm because it keeps their muscle bulk up and the legs look better. Beyond any medical benefits from standing (possible improved skin, bladder, and bone care), and the more subjective personal aspects of standing, LARSI also made the body look in better shape. Julie had spent months doing FES to bulk up her muscles. This had brought her attention back to her body, an area she had neglected or even avoided since her injury.

"To an extent I did see myself after the injury as residing, as having my self, more in my head and body and tailing out in the legs. The LARSI helped that; I am more of a whole body now, because I have that control, because I can move if I want to and because the legs look better. I have more of a sense of whole; before my body stopped at the waist."

If her visible self looked better, then she felt happier about ownership of it. In addition, she seemed to be saying, once she could again determine its movement, then that control and initiation of movement led her to feel more within her body herself. She could decide when and what moved, "albeit electronically, but I pressed the button. I decided to start it, and I decide to start exercising and when to stop. It is all inside, and if you can't see it, it is not there."

I asked if, when she watched others move in sport or at home, how immersed in the movement she became. Julie thought it was similar to before her injury, with "a mirror inside her head" reflecting what she saw. "I can picture myself kicking a ball still."

I wondered to what extent using the LARSI system was similar to this; was she doing it? "Yes, I do feel I am doing it, but it is not complete ownership. On the bike there is a feedback so the bike talks to the box. I have control of the power; I sort of feel both the amount of power the muscles will put in and the amount of effort I put in. Remember, it is hard work and very tiring. My body still works."

"One reason for my resting from FES is that when I start again I am physically ill. I vomit and probably pass out; my body always does that to me, but then it improves. I must admit I have not exercised for a couple of months, but I have had some medical problems. ["Some medical problems": Julie had broken her leg (a clumsy taxi driver), then had a deep vein thrombosis and needed a bladder stone removed.] It all conspired against me, but I will exercise again.[7]

"There have been times, over the years with the LARSI system, when I have almost been trapped into it. I couldn't stop; there were too many people's careers and Ph.D.s hanging on it. Now it is up to me, and maybe now I am not using it because I do not have to. Not having anyone there driving it forward is a relief. Basically they have given up on me now. They will service any part, but there is no more money. I still have the bike, but not at this time of year. And I need to keep the muscles up. It is still there and I will do it."

Me, My, Mine

I came back to her LARSI movements and how much they had become second nature. Her first thought, she had written, when it was turned on was that it was *"My nerves, my muscles, mine."*

"I do not have to put intellectual effort in, but I breathe hard and my heart goes up and I sweat a lot, from the waist up. I am really out of breath. The LARSI uses muscles less efficiently with a slow ramp up and down. It may not look strenuous, but it is. I don't hurt, but the body, my body, says enough."

It must be extraordinary to be out of breath from the effort your body has produced, yet not to have ordered that movement directly yourself. Going for a long arm push in a chair, I thought, Julie would move normally, with perhaps a sense of pleasure and achievement and a sense of connecting with her body. But this would not be the case for a LARSI cycle. When moving her arms, I suggested, she was commanding action, but when using the LARSI not . . .

"But I am deciding when to press the button."

I asked if this makes the LARSI movements more distant than her arm movements. Was the ownership of the two movements similar?

"Equal, I think. My upper body is totally normal and part of me, so I do not think about it. In a way the movement or the ability I have with LARSI, because they should not work at all, is almost special because I can make them work. But it is never an unconscious movement with

LARSI. I am always aware of the process. It is second-hand but it is different. Remember I cannot compare this with anyone, either."

When I kick a ball, I explained, I decide to do it and it happens. I hardly think about what I am doing; that is how action is. When LARSI standing, could she take over the action and make it her own?

"Not really. If it were perfect [i.e., worked better] then I think I could. But standing is always hard, because of the hip problems, etcetera. When I stood with the external FES it was easy and I could stand relaxed, almost with no hands, and just use fingertip control. We hoped for that with LARSI. If that were so I would have more ownership. At its best, when I took steps—I never walked—it was exhilarating, and I had to ask myself why? I had to challenge the feeling, 'Why was it so good?' when it was incredibly hard work. I had, for instance, to look down to see where my feet were.

"I think it was a sense of achievement and the whole science thing, and that it was working and that it was possible. It isn't, wasn't, ever going to be anything more than taking some steps. If it had been more, then great. If it was perfect, then I still do not know how much I would use it, because it is so hard work."

Normally we make movements without thought and retain a sense that they are ours. In more difficult or unusual movements we may have to attend to them, but still our sense of ownership persists. But for Julie, despite her wanting LARSI because its hidden wires made its movements belong more to her, the residual difficulties of movement precluded a merging of her command with the action. It remained, I thought, foreign. But at times, during the first turn-on and at times of triumph she had taken it over. The question was not resolved either way, but an ease and facility of movement seemed necessary to fully own movement.

Mapping Sensation

Enough of her new movements. I was also fascinated by her writing about sensation and how she might know she was being stimulated in areas in which she has no feeling.

"If you touch your hair, you know, but you cannot feel the touch. If I touch my legs I know."

But what if someone else touches them, I asked.

"Then I do not know, unless I see them do it. . . . But then I know they are and I can feel a presence."

I asked about any other sensation from the legs, not necessarily related to touch.

"As I sit here, I can feel like an inner core, with buzzing around the knees and the big toe on left and ankle on the right, and if I concentrate I can transfer those feelings into a sense of legs, my legs, even though slapping on my thigh is nothing."

This buzzing was quite a common experience; I presume it is due to a nonpainful "phantom" sensation after the removal of inputs to the nervous system. It was diffuse and to co-register it onto her body required attention. But in addition, Julie had a sense of touch in her legs dependent on—and maintained by—vision. Her sense of a leg and of a body below the level, and by extension her sense of self and of her body as a whole was, in part, dependent on a visible self, seen in front of her in the chair. Her "sense of touch" on the skin, which was amazingly vivid, seemed dependent on *seeing* that touch in a certain place and then elaborating it from a visual to sensory/tactile experience.

The hair analogy was close, but not exact. Our hair is dead, and dead to the touch—otherwise a haircut would be torture—but when hairs are touched the feeling is transmitted down the hair to the follicle and skin underneath, and that is where we feel. For Julie some sensations might be similar; big movements of her legs and hips might be transmitted to an area above the spinal problem where she could feel, and then projected (nonconsciously) back, or referred, below the level to be "felt." But more than this, she seemed to be suggesting that she transferred seen touch from a visual mode to a cutaneous tactile mode and could elaborate this sufficiently onto and into her seen self so that it was actually felt in the leg. This required attention and was a "top down" way of feeling, which is why she could feel touch only when she saw touch.

I suggested to Julie that she elaborated almost a "phantom touch" felt on the leg via visual perception. This, I suggested, must give more sense of ownership of her body?

"Very much so. It is something I have learned to use over the years, like with sexuality. One consultant had the perception that with complete paralysis from the waist down all I could be was a breeding machine, with no sensation. But, as I said in the book, you can re-map things onto your body, and your mind becomes in tune with it too."

A Good Fag Afterwards

Julie went on to elaborate.

"We have a very good sex life now, because of this retuning. It seems to be from the brain down, it is thought and then down into the body. We had not had an active sex life for ten years before, and now it is better than before. It is now a mind and body thing, rather than just sex.

"I know I get release, and some guys with cord injuries also get release. At one talk, Anne Seaman, a nurse with expertise in sexuality and spinal cord injury, quoted me as saying, 'I know when it has been good because I need a good fag afterwards.' It is hard to quantify, and maybe it should not happen. But it has grown over the years. I am not unique—if you get a group of spinal cord injured women together talking, just like getting any group of women together, then we talk about sex. We are probably more honest than men and do not talk so much of conquests.

"Most people can map some feeling and sensation onto the right bit and get some release. It is a physical thing. Discovering your own sexuality takes some time and it takes time to realize that all this is possible with what you have."

When injured there must be a huge loss, not just of sensation but also of the ability to focus and concentrate on the insentient part of one's body. Then, with the realization that if one concentrates one can find small clues about bowel and bladder sensation and about pressure problems and balance and a myriad of other things, one learns about one's body in new ways. It must take a while longer to realize that some fun things can be mapped onto the body as well.

If sexual pleasure might be so mapped, "top down," I wondered just how one might feel good about one's body and one's self, as this seemed to be the prerequisite for successful sexuality. To an extent sexual desire is body based (though I am aware of gender differences here), and I presumed this is more difficult with a paralyzed and insentient body. It must need an ingenuity to find this within yourself, to find that part you are happy with and can project to others and have them enjoy too. And this may not be confined to sexuality alone.

Julie agreed. "It is individual, and I could not answer for others. Feeling good about yourself, loving yourself and being happy with yourself—that is a tough one. When I first had my accident, I was not happy with myself, I hated myself and my body and all about myself—for two years or so.

"It is having the confidence to go out there, and not being dragged into a mire of disability, and focussing on what you can do, not what you cannot. At some point you have to put to the back of your mind what you cannot do and focus on the positive. It does not always happen to those with spinal injury. You have to step over a bridge and accept what you can do and make the most of what there is; then it does not seem so bad."

Simply said, but this took Julie two years or more before she was ready for an even more difficult problem—putting others at ease. It was far longer, she thinks, before her husband Kevin and some of her friends saw her as a person again. Interestingly, Julie thinks her two sons were far more able to do this, instinctively.

"My boys were four and six when I had the accident, and I think they have grown up to be nicer people because they are aware of disability and what it can cause. They still use and abuse me as kids do—that is not a problem—but they seem to have more empathy and understanding of others."

That led me to ask her just how much one could empathize with being in a chair. Can you know what it is like to be in a wheelchair?

"I am not sure you can. If you have politicians in a wheelchair for just one day, then they would begin to understand and they should rethink about access issues. They think they understand having talked to a few people, but they do not . . . though even being in a wheelchair for a day will not do it, the lack of spontaneity, and more. . . ."

Spontaneity is not solely about doing what one wants at a given time. It is as much about having the confidence to cope with whatever may come up and to enjoy the coping. Young people traveling abroad learn this and much more. Perhaps, I asked, people with tetraplegia might not remember what it was like to walk. Their experience was normal for them now. After all, how do we remember what it is like to be a kid? You cannot remember all of it.

"You just have snapshots. You cannot remember. Spontaneity is the biggest miss for me. When I go to bed, I get next day's clothes near. I shower and do my ablutions at night since it suits me, but I have to plan. If I go out, I have to think of access. I cannot just go. I do miss that. I have to think things through first."

I asked if she could remember what it is like to walk, effortlessly? What it was like to have sand between the toes?

"Snapshots again. But then my memory might not be that different to yours if you had not been on a beach for a while. I still always walk when I dream, sometimes with difficulty. The chair is usually around, and sometimes I push it, and then towards the end of the dream I may get back in it."[8]

Julie always says that she did not and would not chose the injury, but that it has made her a better person and, by extension, has given her family more empathy and insight into others. With their help and that of others she has also seen far more of the world than she would have otherwise.

"My disability has hardly prevented me from doing anything. On the contrary, it has given me a renewed lust for life."

She has begun to make a new career as a counsellor, using an interest in others she was previously unaware of. In this, she feels in one sense more whole now than before. She has a new mission, not to stand again, not to be a "super-para," not to be seen as someone who has achieved so much "despite being disabled." She wants to be good at being her, Julie Hill, just a person like anyone else. Best to agree with her, I thought, because as she says, with the LARSI system she could kick out from the grave.

9

Me and It

At seventeen, after a year of studying the wrong A level courses, Deborah felt it was unlikely she would pass the exams. She moved out of her parents' home to live with her boyfriend ninety miles away. "That," she said, "pissed people off." She found a job in a community for people with autism, which was very rewarding, but stressful and poorly paid. So, after two years and with the romance spent, she decided to become a social worker. She moved back in with her parents and started an access course. She got a job in a bar to make ends meet, and promptly met another man. Soon she moved in with him and, when he was promoted, followed him to South Devon, a few miles down the coast. They both ended up working in holiday parks, and then moved to Weymouth in Dorset. Studying took the back seat for awhile. Soon though, she was restless again, split from her boyfriend and started silkscreen printing, something, at last, which she loved.

She decided to become a primary school teacher (for grades 1–4), and enrolled in a class to gain the qualifications for teacher training college. Life was manageable, though busy, with the course two days a week, the silk screening, and bar work to supplement her income. She was accepted in a teacher-training course in Winchester, a hundred miles to the east, and juggled this with the bar work.

One summer night Deborah and a group of friends were drinking in the Weymouth Holiday Camp when they decided to go swimming and climbed over the pool fence.

"It was 3 a.m. and I did dives between a friend's legs. I thought I would do higher and higher dives, so I got the lifeguard's chair from the side and dragged it to the pool, and dived off that. For my finale I dived from the top of the chair. The pool was not deep and I knew it. So I dived in, missed the bottom, and glided across the pool. Then I hit the other side and broke my neck. I like to be different. I went through the legs as well. It was one of those things. I have seen so many others hit their heads on the side without injury.

"I knew immediately. Maybe I was destined to do it. I could not turn over and, face down, thought I would drown. Luckily I cut my head open at the same time. I could hear people messing around and then my friend said, 'Oh my God, Debs is dead.' They turned me over.

"I had done lifeguard training. I knew I should not be moved. They phoned 999, but when they arrived the ambulance men could not get in since we had climbed over the wall. So they broke the door down and then got in the water. I had been in the pool a long time, and they took me to Weymouth Hospital to warm up. Then I was transferred to the spinal center once warm enough."

The transfer was not uneventful.

"I was quite drunk and was sick a lot, and I remember someone saying it was blue. That would have been the cocktails from the night before.

"I was strapped into the ambulance on a stretcher, and we went slowly to Odstock. I was sick several more times, and could not move my head. They had to stop the ambulance to turn me over to stop me choking. I had long hair and I kept apologizing because it was in my hair. Once in Odstock, just as they got me cleaned up I was sick again. That was grim. Not being able to turn over, they kept having to call the crash team, since each time I was sick I had to be sucked out.

"I don't remember much more. They may have given me something, and thereafter I just lay there."

Deborah had a complete motor level at C5/6 but always had some sensation of touch, though she was unsure of temperature. She remembers feeling the pulse oximeter on her finger they used when she was admitted.

She was in the hospital for nine months and, by the end of it, extremely bored.

"When I came out I was very negative about it, and thought that people could have done more. But now, looking back, I am less critical. Everybody seemed to be emphasizing what I would not be able to do: feed myself, clean my teeth. . . . Most people were not positive. Even the OTs seemed not to be thinking of ideas. So I came up with the ideas. Maybe that was good, since at least I did it—maybe it was designed that way.

"I also felt that I was not told everything. Maybe people get in a groove. They drum into you that you have to look after your skin. So I felt I would not be able to sit in an armchair, since I did not think I could relax in the evening in my wheelchair. In fact in an armchair I am much more comfortable, since I am supported. I can relax and not worry about falling over." Deborah, being C5/C6, has no control of her posture.

"The first time in a wheelchair I felt like I was on a horse with no saddle and no reins. Now to sit in a chair I hook on with my arms round the back of the pushing handles initially, and then I sit straight and balance as best I can. I am still more stable leaning forward with my arms on a table. I also wear jeans, to give a little support in the stomach. I was told not to, but I have found them good. When I came out, I went through all my clothes thinking I would not be able to wear them again. I thought it would be loose tracksuits for the rest of my life. Then I realized that I would be able to wear almost what I liked. I did not feel anyone was particularly interested. Even in physiotherapy I felt they thought, 'Who's going to do the tetraplegics?' You see, with no transfers unaided and no balance, there was little they could do."

This was all over seven years ago, and she has mellowed a little. Talking with her, I asked about her sensation. She was uncertain if what she felt now was because her brain had elaborated or whether it was actually well preserved for touch if not for temperature.

"I have good sensation, I think, though I am motor complete. I don't know if the sensation is good, or my brain is taking over and elaborating. I think I can feel touch, but I cannot feel hot or cold.[1] I can feel a pair of shoes and if my right heel hurts. Thinking about it, I can definitely feel pain and I can get someone to point to where it is."

Quickly I tested light touch and joint position and movement sensation. This appeared very good, though more sophisticated testing would be necessary to say how normal it was.

"When I left hospital I lived with my parents, in a chalet bungalow near the harbor. I was adamant that I would not live at home. But I was so bored in hospital, and though I had a grant to do my house up it was not ready, so I moved in with my parents and thought I could then hurry the builders up. I poached a carer from Odstock to look after me."

I asked whether she called her assistant a carer or personal assistant. Deborah laughed. If she advertised for PAs, she said, she would get secretaries. In the end, Deborah's parents moved to a small street near the town center, and a couple of years later she bought the house next door, when the owner's wife asked for a divorce and needed the money. Deborah is independent, yet has her parents close by. Her dad is the local harbor master and her brother has a boat brokerage business. Deborah and her mother work in the business as well, for fun, and because it makes no money she does not get paid. She does get her supper cooked occasionally, though.

It's Outrageous

"I heard about the Freehand through my Dad. He was doing the bridge at the harbor when a bloke sidled up to him in a wheelchair. My dad was examining him, as you do when you have a daughter in a chair, seeing if he was a para or a tetra, and they got chatting. This man had had a tendon transfer and showed Dad."

A tendon transfer is a surgical procedure in which a muscle is hitched to another tendon, so moving the muscle to act on another joint, or to act in another way at the same joint. Because of the level of a spinal cord injury the muscles that move the arm out at the shoulder might be spared, but those controlling elbow straightening might be paralyzed. A tendon transfer may then allow some return of function below the apparent level of the injury.

"They started comparing levels and completeness, as blokes do. I get blokes come up to me and say, 'I like your wheels, what are they made of? How much do they weigh? What tires you got?' And I don't know at all, they just look nice. Boys and their toys.

"He showed Dad his new grip, and Dad said go in and meet Debs, she would like to meet you. So he came in and introduced himself, and showed me how he could grip and hold a cup. He went over and picked up the kettle, and he could hold a pen and a tablet.

"I thought, 'I want that, why have I not heard of that? It's outrageous.' He said that I only had to ring the hospital to get an appointment.

"So I did, and went to see Mr. Tromans. I said I've met this bloke, and he has it and I want one. I went for an assessment. The surgeon, Mr. Hobby, came in and said I was not suitable, since I did not have sufficient power in lifting the wrist to allow him to halve that power by a tendon transfer. But he did say I would be perfect for a Freehand System. I had heard a little about it but had not gone into it. I thought it was all electronic and not me. I liked the tendon transfer because it would be me and my hand doing it. Not a computer, but me."

"More Spontaneous"

The Freehand System[2] involves placing eight electrodes under the skin of the forearm onto muscles. The wires are connected to a small receiver in the anterior chest wall, under the skin. This is driven by a radio transmitter lying on the skin over the receiver. The transmitter signals are determined in turn by movement of the subject's shoulder via a shoulder position sensor or transducer. Moving the shoulder backwards or forwards allows the hand to open and close. Like this, it sounds simple.

"I went away and found out more. I read a lot and then went to see someone who had it. George and his wife were really positive, especially his wife. She said it had changed his life, and I remember coming away and saying to my parents, who came with me, that I did not feel like I needed to change my life. I don't know what he was like before, but I did not really feel I needed it like that. It gave him far more confidence and allowed him to drive. I had done this and I was not just sitting at home. She was saying that his attitude had changed and he was far more positive.

"It was exciting because I could see his hand moving and working, but on the other hand, I wondered if I was disabled enough. I still don't think it has changed my life, but I do have more independence.

I could do most things before . . . use a telephone, a cup, write, tap at a computer, but I would have to use a splint to do so. I could write, but it was not good. I could not use a hair dryer—I had short hair so I did not need one."

The surgeon was really positive. Deborah spoke on the phone with several others who had the system, and she looked on the Internet. She decided she had little to lose, and that even if she did not gain as much as George, it would be good not to have to use a splint to eat. She was concerned not to get too hyped up about it. Her big hope was really to be a little more spontaneous.

By this time Deborah had a film crew in tow. She had organized a weekend waterskiing in Nottingham, and had enjoyed it so much that she decided to set up a disabled weekend near her. She found some sponsorship, and a local TV company wanted to film it. They made a five-minute feature, and when Deborah mentioned the operation they decided to make a documentary. As it had with Julie, this made it more difficult for her to back out.

First, though, the relevant muscles had to be built up. With the help of her family, Deborah stuck electrodes on the skin over the muscles and stimulated for fifteen minutes to start with, increasing up to four hours per day for three months. Her training was all tailored toward the operation date and then, at the last minute, it had to be postponed from October to February. She was "gutted" and, for a while, stopped the exercises. Then she started again.[3]

Two operations were planned. The Freehand system allowed a grip, but Deborah also needed greater power of elbow extension to allow her to use that grip in a variety of situations. The surgeon decided on a tendon transfer from her strong shoulder muscle deltoid, supplied by nerves above the injury that moved her arm out, to triceps, supplied by damaged cord and so paralyzed and that normally allowed her elbow to straighten. To extend the deltoid muscle from the shoulder to reach the triceps tendon just above the elbow, doctors used a Goretex graft. These operations required periods of immobilization; the Freehand needed three weeks to allow the electrodes to become encapsulated. The tendon transfer required one week in a cast, with six further weeks in a brace, slowly increasing the range of motion by fifteen degrees each week.

New Triceps

The operations went well. Then Deborah had to wait for postoperative healing before trying her new triceps and the new grip. After this she had some new movements, and some new tricks to master. The deltoid, which had previously moved her upper arm outward, now did two things. Half of it still moved her shoulder, but the other half now straightened her elbow. (These two movements are often performed together, with shoulder and elbow moving outwards. But there were also times when the two muscles have differing actions, for instance when the elbow straightens without arm elevation.) But the wiring in her brain was unaltered. How could she move the elbow rather than the shoulder? What would she have to think of? I asked if she had had to think about what movement she had left in a new way. Up to a point, she agreed.

"Before the surgery I just used my hand, without thought. But I did have to think of ways around the weakness. I would not think about a movement but how annoying it was not to pick something up properly. I would lick my fingers to make them sticky, not think about putting more effort into my muscles. I have good wrist extension, so I could always pick up [since extension leads to curled over fingers and a grip of sorts]."

We habitually move with little or no thought. Only when movements become difficult, such as walking over a narrow bridge, or when we are learning a new movement do we expend conscious effort.[4] After her injury, Deborah had to think how to sit in a chair without falling forward, or how to eat. These entailed a mixture of attending to new movements and habits, and finding new ways—tricks—to do things people had thought she might be incapable of doing. The tendon transfer was entirely different. This required her movement brain to adapt from producing a shoulder movement to producing shoulder and, sometimes, elbow movement either together or separately.

"The first time I tried to move, it just did it. It was weird."

This surprised me, so I asked Deborah to reproduce her first new movement. It was a movement of the shoulder outward and backwards, with a straightening movement of the elbow as well. This clearly was not different in motor focus from before, it just led to two movements instead of one.

I wondered what happened when she tried to extend her elbow without shoulder elevation.

"I can compare with my left shoulder, where I have not had a transfer.[5] Since I had the operation, I feel the muscle under my skin and in my arm. Now, doing a different movement to what I should be, I really think about it. I know that actually, in my brain, I need to think about it to make my new triceps work. I think, 'Try to go straight.'"

I asked if she made a motor command for her arm to go straight? She returned to her unoperated on left arm.

"No. When I try to extend my left arm, I know what I want to do, but the message does not get there. . . . I picture it in my arm. I picture the message going from my brain down my spinal cord and coming to a dead end. It does not go further. I know how I should do it, but it does not work. It is like if I try to move my feet. I know the feeling in my brain and I know what I should be thinking, and I occasionally do think it. Not so often now. I did think the other day lying in bed, wouldn't it be weird if I thought about moving my legs and they moved, since I have not thought about moving my legs for such a long time. In my moments of lying in bed, I think I should try to think about moving, in case my brain forgets what it has to do. Otherwise one day I might be able to move but will have forgotten how to."[6]

I returned to her right arm. Did she picture the elbow straightening, or think of the movement?

"I think of the movement. For my right arm, when I lift up my shoulder and my elbow extends, that is relatively easy. But when I want to extend the elbow without shoulder movement, then it is not easy. Sometimes, say in bed, gravity helps to flop my elbow out. But say, if in bed with my arm on my stomach, to straighten it then I use the new triceps alone. Moving my shoulder I don't think about, but using the new triceps I do. Then I think about pushing my arm out. The new muscle feels as though there is an elastic band inside the arm.

"I get the thought to the right muscle because of this band in my arm. They took the plaster off after three weeks. The new triceps felt like a tight elastic band [because of the implanted Goretex graft]. I moved, and as I moved it felt as though the band was tighter. Now I don't feel that it's the same message that I used to send, because it is a different muscle. I don't feel like it was before my accident. Maybe because I have to think about it still, nineteen months after the operation. I do not have to think about deltoid movement and new triceps at the same time, but for new triceps alone I do, because it is not natural. It feels like a pull in the arm."

So, I wondered, what if I asked her to move her deltoid and new triceps together and then I suddenly prevented elbow but not shoulder movement?

"I would immediately feel the resistance. I can feel it working in my arm and I know what it is. I don't feel deltoid."

It seemed that initially she might have made the same motor command as before, but that the sensory return from movement was odd (not shoulder abduction but elbow extension). This unexpected feedback from the periphery, possibly from the old triceps tendon to which the deltoid was connected, and due to new sensation within the upper arm, alerted her to what was happening. She agreed.

"If I do not think about it, then I cannot do it. I am not thinking about a picture of my arm. I am thinking about making that muscle work. I am thinking I must make the muscle move to make my arm go straight. If I flex my biceps or deltoid, then I am not thinking."

The tendon transfer seemed complicated enough. But next I asked about using the Freehand itself.

Freehand/Frankenstein

"When I first used the Freehand, it was weird. I had used the surface stimulation and then I could feel the buzzing from the electrodes on the skin. With the Freehand, when I switched it on, I initially could not feel it, and so I felt like Frankenstein. The surface stimulation I had controlled, whereas with the Freehand the electronics engineer switched on. It felt like a computer was controlling my hand, which is what it was.

"Then I became aware of the stimulation—a buzzing, but not painful. Before I could feel it on the outside, whereas now, with the Freehand, I felt it under my skin. The muscles felt a little as though they were waking up, with the sensation coming from inside. I was surprised there was still muscle there that worked."

These muscles, activated by the internal device, were the same ones that had been activated for months through the external electrodes.

Now the internal buzzing and the absence of external devices allowed her to think of her muscles awakening.

There are eight electrodes, four on different muscles in the forearm that control her finger flexors and extensors, and four on the thumb muscles for normal movement of the thumb.[7] Wrist extension is under voluntary control, though it too has been strengthened by a tendon transfer. The system locks the position of her hand, not her wrist. As her fingers flex with use of the Freehand, this pulls her wrist into flexion, which she has to resist herself. With the mixture of Freehand movement and its buzzing and her various tendon transfers for wrist and shoulder it is not surprising that she finds it difficult to be sure what she does and what the machine does.

She showed me the combined effect of Freehand and her, with two grips, one with the thumb opposed and one not. One allows a fine grip for holding a fork or writing, whereas the other is a coarser grip for larger, heavy objects, such as Deborah's hair dryer. Though initially she found the decision to have the procedure difficult, once it was working it was, simply, "brilliant."

She turned on the Freehand and showed me her fingers locked in flexion, or mid extension, by various shoulder movements, with her fingers gripping, with the thumb opposed or not.

"To use my Freehand [on the right] I have to move my left shoulder. To pick a pen up, I first position the pen in front of me, then I put my left arm around the back of the chair to stop falling over. I switch the system on by pressing a button on my chest, and then I pull my left shoulder back and the right wrist is extended and the hand open. Then as I move the shoulder forward—slowly and a very small amount—the wrist and hand close. Small opposite movements will open and close the hand.

"The shoulder movement is forward and back. Once my hand is gripping as I want, I flick my shoulder suddenly, and it locks the system. Then I can hold with my clenched hand, without thought, and move my shoulder independently. When I want to release my hand, I flick the shoulder again and the hand relaxes. Then I switch it off by pressing again."

Deborah showed me this several times. It looked a little like she was using her hand and wrist as a mole wrench. Once her hand was gripping the pen satisfactorily, she clamped the hand and could move the forearm and hand by more proximal movements, with the knowledge that nothing short of power failure would release the fixed positions of her fingers and hand.

"I cannot feel it doing anything on the muscles, except a little when it is locked. It feels as if there is a current in my arm. I don't feel the contracting muscles, but this is partly because I can feel the current as a buzz that gets in the way. I can feel my fingers when they are digging into my palm, since that is painful. Otherwise I can just feel my fingertips, but not their movement, because this is obscured by the buzz. But I would still know about finger position a little because there would be different buzzing. When my hand is open, the buzzing is less than when closed."

She learned to use it through a sophisticated process of trial and error. At Odstock, an engineer and a physiotherapist would switch on the various channels for various shoulder movements, and together she and they explored the level of muscle activation and left shoulder movement sufficient to hold something. This needed a lot of fine-tuning. Occasionally she still moves too far and the contraction is too strong. It is so complicated that it is a long way from being "second nature"—she always thinks about it as she does it.

"I always know what I am going to do. I decide to make a movement. Coming back to the pen, I start with it in position and then get the hand open with the Freehand, and then, by small movements, I will get the optimum position. Then I lock my hand by flicking the shoulder quickly. Then I know I must not move my shoulder or it would unlock. So I cannot shrug my shoulders.[8]

"I look at my hand, but think about my shoulder. I am not in any way thinking about muscles in arm or hand or about muscles in my shoulder, I am thinking about moving my shoulder and about getting the pen in the right place visually. Once locked, I still have to write from my whole arm, since I cannot use my fingers—they are locked—so my writing is still not what I would like. But it is easier than before, because I have a proper grip.

"Before, I could not press down or the pen would come out of my hand. To write I think about the whole arm. Before, or without the Freehand, I would focus on the hand. [She can always decide to use it or not.] I cannot really think about anything else. I have to hold my breath. I do really. I think about writing neatly."

She showed me by writing her name again and again on a piece of paper, both with and without using the Freehand. Without, her writing was faint on the page and a little wobbly. With it, the script was clearer and firmer, though still recognizably the same handwriting.

"Without the Freehand I would have to think about sitting up so I am hooked over and not likely to fall. Then I have to hold my arm up in the air to get some weight behind it. All I am thinking about is writing. With the Freehand on, I think about the grip and then lock it, and after that all I am thinking about is the neatness of the writing. And I can talk and breathe at the same time, though I prefer not to speak. I still have to think about sitting and balance. But I don't have to think quite so much about sitting up, because the Freehand means I can lean forward on the table."

I wondered about a grasping or holding movement.

"I set up the shoulder and the Freehand grip. Then I don't have to think about the movement. Then I can think about the action and its goal. Once locked, that is the job done, the hand locked for the hair-brush. The Freehand is my tool for the grip, and then once set up I set about the goal. I get the hair dryer in the right place so it will not fall out of my hand, and then I get on with the job.

"If I am on the phone at my brother's boat business, then that is slightly harder, since I am holding the phone with my left hand, with a hook on the back of the handset for my fingers, and trying to type a name with my right hand locked by the Freehand. I have got a metal pen with a rubber to type with. I am then careful not to move my shoulder and to sit up, and I also lean onto my left elbow to give me the stability to type. If I want to put phone down, I say 'Goodbye,' and put the phone down, and then I can unlock the hand by jerking the shoulder. And I am thinking mainly about getting his name right."

"Slightly harder," I thought, seemed an understatement. Answering the phone for her was more complicated than most people's movements in their daily lives. Deborah was doing it from a chair with a combination of tendon transfer, Freehand system, balance, and determination—coupled with a mental concentration upon various movements of trunk, shoulder, and arm. Living from a wheelchair may look passive and devoid of action, but that is far from the truth. I could well imagine that learning to use the Freehand system took a while. I wondered if it was more automatic now, nearly two years on?

"First I thought about the system more than the goal. When I used it to pick up a fork, my attention was more on the shoulder movement and the fork's position in my grip than in using the fork to eat. My attention is now more on the action, and less on the hand. It is now more on what I am doing, though of course when the system is not locked my attention is on setting up. My attention is now more to the hand and the goal; when I was learning, it was more on the shoulder. I attend the object now."[9]

I had thought initially that she might use the Freehand to move, but it had become clear that she used it to lock into a position, which then allowed her to use the hand through movements more proximally in the arm. "I don't really move with the Freehand, I set up movements and then make them myself."

I was interested in how much this allowed her to consider the hand and its movements hers or not. It was evident that this is difficult for her to answer, because she still does not feel completely in control of the system.

"When I do control it, then it becomes me. Well, kind of me. When it is not working, then it is the stupid bloody thing. When it is working, it is me, since I am controlling it through my shoulder. But I do look at my hand differently when using the Freehand system. It is still not completely me, still alien, still something else, since it is being controlled by a computer in a bag on the back of my chair. Without the Freehand, it is me completely, even though I cannot move it well. When it works, it is the system and me controlling the system, but still not me completely.

"And I do not completely own it because it can dig my fingers into my hand. . . . I say 'it'. . . . though it is my fingers digging in, I am not in control of them, so it is 'it' doing it. If I were in complete control, then it would be me.

"So when it is doing something I want to, like writing, it is me, and when it is doing something I do not want exactly, then it is 'it.'"

This was in part jocular, but also deeply within her. When it did what she wanted when she wanted it, when it behaved like her shoulder and as normal, then it became more her, more herself embodied. When command and action were as one, then "it" was her.

"I own it once locked on and once I control it. But even then I can never quite forget the computer, and it never allows you to do exactly what you want, so there is always a compromise. Control is inadequate, despite the brilliant setting up. Don't forget also that it is my hand, but there is a current going through it making it move, which I can always feel."

By now Deborah was anticipating my next question. "If you moved my hand and compared it with movement via the Freehand, it would be completely different, since I would know what I was doing and going to do next with the Freehand, but not what you were doing."

A crucial indicator of the success of any device is how often it is used in daily living. This tells when the bother is worth it.

"I use it depending on what I am doing. During a normal day I use it when I brush my hair. My PA dresses me, and anyway the computer is too big on my chair for it to be useful for me in dressing. It would be too hard anyway. If at home, I would use it for eating, writing, and doing my hair. In the shop I use it all the time to write. At home I may use it to put a video in. It can be fun to use, to see if I can open the fridge or cook a potato in the oven. I also find increasingly that I go to prepare a grip with my shoulder even when I have not connected the Freehand."

I mentioned a robot at NASA. There is a set of markers and position sensors on your arms that control movement of the robot's arms. You see the robot arms through a 'virtual reality' set. Within a few minutes of moving your arms—but seeing the robot's arms move and with your focus on the goal of moving the robot arms—you are completely embodied in the robot.[10] More than that, the use of the robot is strangely fascinating and absorbing, and indeed outright fun. I hoped the Freehand gave some fun in movement too, especially when setting it up. I asked about becoming embodied in a hand seen by her, that was her, but moved by the Freehand system.

"Now I come to think of it, maybe. . . . I am not quite sure. Now I think about the robot hands, then maybe I am not completely in control of the Freehand, since I cannot make it do what I want, but maybe with the Freehand I can do more. So which is more me?

"Using the system, setting it up, it is not me, since I have to think about it and need to move my shoulder. But once it is set up, it becomes more me again. I do find myself talking to my hand when I try to pick something up. If it opens when I want to pick something up, I look at it and talk to it and say, 'Pick it up.' Then I am not thinking of my shoulder but of my hand doing what I want. As I bring it under control, then it becomes more me, and I can eat. When it does not do what I want, it is not me. I am not thinking about my left shoulder. My attention is to my right hand not doing what it should be, but not about the shoulder, for a nanosecond or so."

It seemed that Deborah's attention was split between hand and shoulder when setting up and went from one to the other, depending on which part of the Freehand maneuver she was engaged in and how well it was going. With more familiarity, the focus had moved from shoulder to hand and then, perhaps, from hand to goal. Then once the hand was clamped, her focus moved to her proximal arm muscles and to writing neatly.

"I love the Freehand system, though I am annoyed because it does not always work properly. It is scary that before my life was perfectly fine and I got on with splints. Now I don't have to use splints, but in the back of my mind I think if it goes wrong I may have to go back to the splints, and that is depressing."

I returned to her new triceps and asked if she could compare this with her new grip. For new triceps action she thinks about it when moving and using it, whereas with the Freehand system she has to think about it as she sets up a movement, but then once set up and the clamp is on her movements may occur with less thought. She agreed, sort of.

"You would think having a tendon transfer and having to physically think about it in use would make it less 'me' than the Freehand system where I do not have to think about it once it is being used. The tendon transfer is just me using me. The Freehand is not me, but I don't have to think about it while I do things which are me with my hand."

By now Deborah was itching to go out for a "gallivant around, looking at nice things to eat." Also, she said, her brain ached. To be honest, mine did a bit, too.

10   Experimentation

Being Upright

Few things illustrate the fundamental shift in perspective that occurs after spinal cord injury more than walking and standing. For most able-bodied people, walking is what people in wheelchairs are missing, and what they most need. But being in a chair also precludes being upright, which society assigns its own values and rewards.

Kay Toombs discusses it thus: "The value assigned to upright posture should not be underestimated when considering the experience of illness. To be able to 'stand on one's own two feet' is of more than figurative significance. Verticality is directly related to autonomy. Just as the infant's sense of autonomy and independence are enhanced by the development of the ability to maintain and upright posture . . . so there is a corresponding loss of autonomy which accompanies the loss of uprightness."[1]

She describes the cultural uses of walking as a metaphor for strength and power, in terms of looking up to and down on, and to work that showed the time a doctor spent with patients is perceived to increase if he sits down with the patient on their bed rather than peers at them from beside it, looking down, even though the actual time is the same. Michael Oliver also suggests that walking is not simply a locomotor act but a symbolic and cultural one. Popular songs stress this: "Something in the way she walks . . .", "Walk Tall," and "He walks like an angel . . ." for example. Oliver's personal favorite is Kenny Rogers' hit, "Don't Take Your Love to Town," with its killer line, "It's hard to love a man whose legs are bent and paralyzed."[2]

Upright posture does not only allow and imply independent movement and eye-to-eye contact; it enables a richness of gesture and of non-verbal communication. Without the freedom to move as we talk and to gesture, either when standing or even sitting, our very style and presentation of self to others is altered and impoverished. One tetraplegic told me of how he feels able to talk to people far more equally when everyone is sitting. Parties, when everyone else is standing, are a trial, especially if he is handed a drink, because then he has no free hand to use to move his wheelchair.

If verticality affects our interactions with others, then does it also affect our relationships with our immediate surroundings? We experience the physical space around us in relation to our own bodies and the potential for movement through that space. Merleau-Ponty writes, "Besides the physical and geometrical distance which stands between myself and all things, a 'lived' distance binds me to things which count and exist for me. . . . This distance measures the 'scope' of my life at every moment."[3]

Toombs takes this up by discussing how illness changes the character of lived space. A narrow doorway becomes a problem rather than being a simple passage. Normal movement opens up space and allows free exploration of new areas and new relations between one's body and the world, so illness and disease limits these potentialities. A bathroom that was near may now be difficult to reach, objects above a certain height unreachable. Toombs, who herself lives from a chair, relates how her first impression of the Lincoln Memorial was not "awe at its architectural beauty, but rather dismay at the number of steps."

She also makes the point that the limitations of movement change not only the way she experiences space and distance, but also time. Whereas we might normally walk from one place to another admiring the view, chatting, or looking at the girls while thinking about the next thing to do, when movement becomes problematic it requires our constant attention and so roots us in the present. Our lives may become a succession of difficult presents rather than a mix of past, present, and future.

That able-bodied people should sympathize with those in wheelchairs about their loss is understandable, even if many aspects of this loss are not really understood. Yet for Colin and for many others, walking may be less important than continence and pain. Despite all the limitations of wheelchair life, walking may not be the big problem, as long as (and this is a very large "as long as") people in wheelchairs have access to where they want and need to go.

Julie Hill seized the possibility of the LARSI trial not to walk, nor even particularly to stand for its own sake; she did it because it allowed her possibilities otherwise denied.

"I would always say this will not replace the wheelchair, but it has given me a choice. I would be like a parrot saying it. 'If I don't stand up then I won't but I could if I wanted: it is my choice.' Walking is not the be all and end all. It is too bloody hard and difficult, and what is the point? I am very able in my chair."

Another very important aspect of the whole project for her was the chance of exercising her body and of exposing it once more to the force of gravity when upright.[4] This is likely to have effects on bone mass, long-term cardiovascular health, and skin durability. Not least, it also allowed her to feel good about her body and her self and, gradually, to feel once more that she inhabited her whole body.

Deborah's Freehand system has, at first look, much more modest purposes, to improve grip and use of the hand. Deborah herself questioned if she needed it, given her comparatively good functioning. I allowed her to use a hairbrush and so grow her hair. But it also allowed her to take down messages at work and so go out into the world. For others, return of some hand function has led to an altered relationship with the world, and to renewed confidence. A comparatively small increase in motor skills can have profound consequences for a given individual.

Owning Movement

Immediately after her injury, Julie spent hours trying to move, trying to reconnect in some way with her body below the injury. "Perhaps through sheer will and bloody-minded determination I could make them move again. It was several days before I realized it was pointless."[5]

Julie's stimulation promised standing and, with this, perhaps enhanced health. But these systems actually promised more than movements alone; they gave the possibility of some reconnection between thought processes and muscles, to allow Julie and Deborah to command movement themselves once more.

The question therefore arises as to the extent to which these movements are similar to natural movements. The conditions necessary for FES to be felt as a reconnection emerged from talking with Julie and Deborah. For both, the sheer difficulties in using the systems precluded them becoming perceptually transparent to them, as our bodies usually are. Julie described just how difficult it was to balance upright with the LARSI, let alone take a step or two, and that unless it became easier it would never become part of her. There was a similar experience with the Freehand. Even though it was smaller and designed to give a simple, useful grip, the fact that it was quite difficult to set up and then had a background buzz meant that Deborah did not really feel it as a part of herself, even when it was working smoothly. These devices need to be so easy to use that their users forget they are actually using them. It was not trivial when Deborah said that when the Freehand was working it was more her and when not working, it.

Echoes of Sensation

One of Julie's first thoughts after her injury was that the ambulance men would see her with legs immodestly up in the air. Such early sensory illusions or hallucinations after sudden loss of sensory input are well known in spinal cord injury and in other sensory losses. Christopher Reeve describes something similar in the days after his injury:

As I started to face reality during the month in intensive care and six months in rehab, moments from my former life kept popping into my head. It was like a slide show, but the pictures were all out of sequence, as if they had been placed randomly in the projector. As a long plastic tube was inserted through my neck and pushed down into my lungs to remove accumulating fluid, suddenly I would be sailing in Maine. But before the next slide appeared on the screen in my mind, secretions were being suctioned up the tube. A moment or two later, Dana and I were making love; I was on a horse jumping over stone walls in the countryside; I was taking a curtain call after a performance in the theatre; carrying boxes and lugging furniture up four flights of stairs into my first apartment in New York. . . .

[Later] more images flashed onto the screen, usually snapshots of my most cherished memories when I was whole and healthy and free.[6]

The most widely known "hallucinations" after sensory losses of various sorts are phantom limb perceptions after loss of an arm or leg.[7] Such formed experiences do, however, seem to appear a little later and to last longer than these present hallucinations. Curiously, those with sensory loss in spinal cord injury rarely say they have vivid and lasting sensory phantoms.[8]

In sudden visual loss there can be a somewhat similar experience in which formed visual hallucinations occur in the hours and days after blindness. In this situation, known as Charles Bonnet syndrome, patients may see geometrical shapes such as bricks, which may reflect activity in a visual cortex once deprived of input. Sometimes more formed images of faces or places may be seen, which may reflect activity in higher cortical areas.[9-11] Whether the later and more formed sensory experience such as Reeve's are the sensory equivalent of Charles Bonnet syndrome remains unclear.

It would be of interest to know whether Reeve's hallucinations were primarily visual, so that he "saw" himself from the outside sailing and moving apartments, or whether his experiences had more of a submerged, first person, sensory and motor aspect. He writes of "moments, like slides." Of course, vision, tactile sensation, and movement are closely interrelated, but one hopes Christopher Reeve's memories had a sensory embodied component and were more than visually replayed experiences.

Both Charles Bonnet syndrome and the hallucinations after spinal cord injury fade within days or weeks, to months. They therefore differ from say, tinnitus, which can follow hearing loss and last for months and years and, of course, from phantom limb pain, which tends to continue once it has emerged. Phantom limb or "deafferentation" pain, so called because it follows loss of sensory input to the brain and spinal cord, is a huge problem after spinal cord injury. The timing of its emergence and its duration suggest that it may result from a slower plastic change within the brain than these early unmasking phenomena that so concerned Julie when the ambulance men arrived.

Seeing Touch

Tactile sensation and vision are not usually thought of as overlapping. In fact, synaesthesia apart, where people have strong visual images with, say, hearing words,[12,13] it seems important to preserve the separateness of the channels between sensory modalities. To see a touch, and then to feel it, would confuse.

Several of those with complete spinal cord injury and serious sensory loss volunteered that they knew where their legs and bodies were despite having no sensation. One woman I saw, with no sensation of touch or position sense below the neck but with deafferentation pain, said that she knew where her legs were. On questioning her, this seemed to be on the basis of two differing mechanisms. It appeared that she spent her life with her body and limbs in one or two positions, in her chair or in bed. She used her vision and a long-term knowledge of where her legs were—in front of her on the chair—to "know" where they were. So strong were these feelings, so strong the illusion that she had peripheral feedback of this in some way, that she was surprised when I convinced her how she made that perception on the basis, essentially, of vision and habit.

In contrast, Julie, despite a lack of touch sensation from the legs, "felt" touch on the thigh when she saw it, and felt when the LARSI system was moving her leg. These may have slightly different origins. She may have felt the sensation of stimulation above the deafferentation area, or her spinal cord injury, as often happens, might not be complete, or some sensation may have reached her brain from nerves going with the intact cranial nerve that supplies the abdominal viscera. More surprising was her vivid sensation of touch on the leg when she saw that touch, but not when she did not see it. Here another mechanism may have been involved.

Quite why they did the experiment is a little unclear, but Botvinick and Cohen placed a rubber hand over their own and then started to stroke the dummy hand.[14] After a few minutes, the subjects began to feel the stroking in their own hands. They had experienced a "visual capture" of the tactile sensation. Since then a large literature on this "cross modality" or multimodality sensory integration has been published,[15] and it has been shown that the dummy hand does not actually have to be realistic for the touch to be felt—a rubber glove works as well.[16]

This is not as counterintuitive as one might imagine. In everyday life, we are constantly engaged in tasks in which sensory modalities affect and influence one another. We sometimes misjudge the weights of objects on the basis of their visible size; we assume a large object is heavier than a light one. The different sensory inputs may be separate on their way to the brain, but as they are made into perceptions, their purity may be compromised.

So the feeling of touch that Julie and others relate on seeing visual touch in an insentient area may reflect a heightened form of visual capture. One might imagine that without sensory input to the sensory cortex, visual inputs would become more dominant. If this occurs while watching a rubber glove being stroked for a few minutes in control subjects, then it may also occur in those who live with spinal injury. Possibly Julie was feeling touch in such a top-down manner, by seeing it first and then elaborating a touch sensation. She agreed, and also realized that without vision she was lost. "Top down describes it well. Sat on the shower chair with my eyes shut, I don't know where anything is until I open them again."

Once she could see her leg, then she could feel it being touched.

Seeing Self

Vision of the body not only gives welcome sensation in an otherwise insentient limb. It is through vision that we see our bodies as others see them, and through vision that we gain some perception of our body image, those feelings and perceptions of our embodied selves. It is through vision, to a significant amount, that we project our selves into the world, and especially project ourselves to the opposite sex. Julie described her feeling thus early on. "Catching a glimpse of myself in a full length mirror . . . the broken body, slumped in the ugly apparatus which was to be my outer skin for the rest of my life. . . . My self esteem hit rock bottom."

Jenny Morris found in her work with women with spinal injury that the altered body image is one of the hardest things to come to terms with. Like it or not, appearance is an important part of our relation with others.[17] More than this, for women (and to an extent men), physical appearance is an important part of femininity (and masculinity) and sexuality. The women Morris interviewed described their experiences thus: "Many of the painful emotions experienced in the months after injury are related to changed body image. We have to get used to a different body." "I cried the first time I saw my skinny body." Another hated her body. "Muscley arms and broad shoulders, a fat stomach and twig like legs. Yuk!"

"I have my tube-shaped muscle-less legs and swollen ankles; my fat abdomen and my tendency to hunch up in the wheelchair." "YES!! The body beautiful image makes me feel bitter and resentful."

"I try hard to accept my body . . . but it's a losing battle. I'm bombarded with pictures of beautiful bodies. I hide my flaws."

Their problems were not just in physical appearance. Several appreciated that they were impoverished in another way. "Body language from the upper chest is limited. And limiting. Friendship gestures toward either sex are now clumsy and awkward instead of natural and fluid."

Without fluidity there was an alteration in the act and the entire experience. Fortunately, the women who spoke with Morris found ways of living with their altered bodies and altered selves. They learned to value themselves and others as people, not just for their appearance. They began to realize that no one is perfect, walking or not. Such changes in perception and attitude were extraordinarily difficult to negotiate or describe, but so important, for despite their efforts, they could not completely divorce self-esteem from their bodies.

With Time and Creativity

One of the most embodied aspects of life seemed to be sexuality. The problems of working around this seemed for some insuperable. Colin had said that "The desire is still there . . . with no release. . . . The inability to reach orgasm and to ejaculate and the absence of that overwhelming sensation of pleasure and release afterward is something I never, ever have got over. I don't think anyone who is able bodied and has experienced orgasm can understand what it must be like not to experience it."

And this is not simply for men. One of Morris's female interviewees had said, "To be totally honest, sex is one thing that torments me more than any other aspect of paralysis. In fact, for me, it has taken over my life as a constant obsession. A person without sexual feelings cannot be normal."

A psychologist told me that he ran a sexuality class for young male spinal cord injured in-patients, which soon got graphic and raunchy.[18] Their drive certainly seemed intact. I asked Anne Seaman, who takes classes in sexuality and sex in spinal cord injury, how some enjoyment might be regained, when often the genitalia are insentient and the capacity to move may be severely reduced.[19] Her answers were similar to those Julie had mentioned, that with time and with creativity, sexual relations can be entered into and enjoyed once more. The person first had to discover ways to find something in themselves that she or he liked and wanted to share.

She also raised how personal these issues are for many clients with an injury, and even for some staff. She thought that for many their return to sexuality occurred after they had been discharged from the hospital, not simply because the ward was a difficult place for such issues, but because of the passage of time. "They grow into it later, and it is not initially a priority. Once discharged, they will do one thing at a time; one year for the house, then another for a holiday, and then they might consider their sexual relations."

Much depended on the age and experience of the individual. Talking with a seventeen-year-old who had never experienced sex was quite different than talking with a mature man or woman. The ones with experience could be more challenging, because they knew what they had lost, but they also knew something about relationships. It was also obviously easier if one was in a relationship at the time of the injury. The key appeared to be, for Anne at least, to leave everything behind and to rebuild this part of their lives from scratch as new. She also made the point that not everyone has a sex life anyway, or even a partner, from choice rather than necessity.

I mentioned to Anne John Hockenberry's observation that those with paraplegia had working upper abdominal muscles and strong arms, so they were seen on the basketball courts, but that they had destroyed the spinal cord and nerves controlling continence and erection.[20] In contrast, the tetraplegics had little motor control, but did have a cord intact enough for reflex erection and ejaculation, and so got all the dates. Anne was slightly appalled.[21] She suggested instead that a woman might see a tetraplegic as being more vulnerable and more in need of her, and in need of comfort and bolstering of his confidence. The size of his possible erection was not part of it. But the guys on the ward were often concerned, once over their acute injury, to leave the wards and hit the pubs to try out their new bodies if they could. For Anne, this had much to do with confidence in one's self and one's body.

Men, she suggested, are more naturally confident and able to project themselves, and need to see if they can still "pull." Yet women have the props of makeup and dress with which to bolster confidence. Some men may go the other way and stop caring for themselves, and not make the best of what they have. Anne described two young lads who went to their first dance after their injuries and returned to the ward devastated that their previous charm and pulling power had gone.

It still seems the case that women with spinal cord injury may get a bad deal. They are outnumbered something like 8 or 9 to 1, so hospital services are skewed toward men. They may also find it difficult to find a partner. Women are for many reasons more likely to be attracted to a neurologically impaired man than vice versa.[22]

I Save That

Anne was less pessimistic about sexuality in the longer term and thought that, for some, orgasm might eventually return in some form after injury. In her survey of women after spinal injury, Jenny Morris found the same.[23] One woman had suggested, "Don't let anyone put you off. Slowly and patiently you and your partner should explore your body: know where your hands are . . . know how and where he is touching you, and enjoy the fantastic sensations. No feeling does not equate to no sensation. Explore all possible erogenous zones. . . . It is not about how often you make love, how often you achieve orgasm, it is enjoying your own body and your partners."

Orgasm can come from other places and in other ways than before. There are many anecdotal reports of areas above the injury becoming remapped as an area for such gratification. Anne remembers touching one man with tetraplegia on the neck during a conversation. He said simply, but unmistakably, "I save that." It may not be orgasm as before, but with patience and attention something can be reinvented and enjoyed, not as simply a memory, but as something of itself.

A woman talking with Jenny Morris related her experience: "I am fairly sure I get what are called 'phantom orgasms,' and we are always game to try new experiments. We use mouth and nose and facial stroking a great deal. . . . We both get turned on by these things and we culminate with my husband entering me. I am very ticklish and can get an orgasm from being stroked under the arms. Love is wonderful stuff and transcends just about everything."

Anne continued. "People have to find out for themselves. They have to look for it and find it. Maybe it is very different for those who have it, and a memory, and those who have never had it. For orgasm, I say you have to work at it. They do understand their own bodies far more than normal people. There is no manual. Rebuild your own confidence."

It is also the case that pleasure from making love becomes as much about turning on one's partner as from oneself—in fact the two become as one. One man described his experiences, and talked for two hours without mentioning his own pleasure. He got his pleasure from his partner, and wanted her to reach orgasm. In a recent survey of fifty men, with a mean of twenty-five years since injury, the predictors of good sexual adjustment and satisfaction were partner satisfaction and relationship quality.[24] What seems important is for people to have the confidence, time, and relationship to explore these things. One woman related how a doctor had suggested that three-quarters of marriages break up, so best get rid of the double bed.

In fact, the figures from marriages do not bear the doctor out. In Morris's sample of 205, sixty-six were single at the time of their injury and twenty have married. Of those 102 who were married, seventy-three still were, with twelve widowed. Figures from the United States suggest that divorce is 2.3 times more common after the first three years of injury. The stressors were complex, involving the reduced ability to homemake, problems with work, childcare, mobility, and finance, as well as psychological adjustment and sexual functioning. Among those that are single, there is a reduced rate of marriage in the first three years, but after that the rate increases and marriages after injury do rather better than those before.[25] Although undoubtedly there can be huge problems in sexuality after spinal injury, some people find ways of experimenting and enjoying this as they do other facets of their lives.

Ian's first thoughts on waking up were, understandably, about what he could not do. Within a few months, his thoughts were about others and about keeping a relationship quiet. For Julie and for Deborah, functional electrical stimulation increased their choices and allowed more involvement with family and more independence. Stimulation for both allowed them to feel that they inhabit and control their physical bodies a little more, no longer petering out in the lower body or arms. In this use of FES, as well as in the reexplorations of sexuality, are seen the self's desire for its body.

Thus far we have concentrated, not surprisingly, on the effects of spinal cord injury on the person injured. But, as we suggested at the beginning, neurological impairment never affects one person in isolation from others. In the next two chapters are reflections of the wife and husband of people who have been through spinal injury. In the first, Rachel and Bob discuss his spinal cord injury and its effects on his life and on their relationship. In the second, Kevin Hill, Julie's husband, gives his side of her—their—story.

V

Observing

11

The Windsurfer

To consider the experience of spinal cord injury in isolation is illusory; each person has a different experience and response. The immediate shock and acute illness are so different from the long rehabilitation and reassembling of life. It is not isolated either in the sense that, though it happens to one person, its consequences affect others too. Thus far our perspective has been from the person with the injury alone. Yet similar adaptations and alterations are necessary for the family and loved ones of the person injured. After the acute period, the tetraplegic has months sheltered from the world as he or she learns new skills. In contrast, the wife or husband has to cope with work and family as best they can.

When the patient comes home after maybe a year away, the family has to rebuild and reacquaint itself with a person whose view of themselves may have altered dramatically. In the next two accounts we will consider what happened next in two individuals, one of whom we have met before.

A Simple Story

Bob had invited me over and then suggested I talk with his wife as well. Rachel would turn up later, Bob said, as he started.

"My story is simple. Had a bad accident. [His wife Rachel later told me it was a car crash.] The next three to four weeks are a drug haze.

I can remember the dreams—they remain vivid: a French gendarme guarding a shipment of gold bullion in a lift, which moved horizontally; a cruise ship that was pirated."

His fracture was at C5/6 and unstable, so he needed a spinal fusion in France. By the time he came to in England he could feel around his shoulder but nothing below. He also had a little leg movement. He was sure, even then, that he would windsurf again. In the hospital, the therapists encouraged and supported, though they worked at too slow a pace for Bob and he always wanted more. In the end he had walked out—just—and seemed puzzled as to why some manage this but not others.

"I accept that some are not going to get better. But some people, like me, can walk out. A young man opposite me in a bed with exactly the same injury as me did not. Two of us got this guy along to show him he could recover . . . but he did not."

It is a difficult thing to understand why some make it and some don't—the damage of an injury does not show on scans and involves not only the direct pressure of a blow, but also swelling and derangement of blood vessels leading to ischemia. This swelling makes it difficult to give a prognosis for some time. Some people may have very similar injuries when they came into hospital and then have very different recoveries, independent of motivation.

Bob left the hospital on crutches. "And I had to fight for those. They said I'd be no good on them. But I knew that I would. I am cynical about medicine. The mind is what determines things. I am a survivor."

For him walking was all.

"I found that they were trying to turn people into a wheelchair existence. I would rather be the world's worst person on a crutch than be in a wheelchair."

I suggested that many people are fine in a wheelchair. Bob was silent. He had been in the services and then, later, a company director. Always very fit. The loss of ease with his body and pride in it was clearly still devastating.

"I was twelve stone of pure muscle in the army. I was always in good shape. Considering what my body has been through it is holding up well. I am not keen on exposing it now. I have lost so much weight. I don't like the change."

The other problem was disordered sensation.

"Though I know where my limbs are, with my right leg I have to watch the lie of the land and I have to watch where I place it. I may think there are two inches to go and there are not. I still have to think about walking the whole time. It is not subconscious as it was. Walking gives me independence. I cannot push a wheelchair because my arm muscles are too weak. But I can walk, after a fashion."

Three Days Out of Seven

It was clear that he was not only weak, but he had also lost some position and movement sensation and, with imperfect knowledge of where his leg was, found walking very difficult. But even this was bearable. Sensation from the skin had been scrambled.[1] Worse was the pain.

"I can put my feet in water and I know it's wet, but I can't be sure if it is hot or cold. I am hypersensitive to touch. A light touch burns and more firm pressure is kinder. Just getting dressed can be a trial, since it is painful. Clothes can also hurt. Putting them on especially. You get used to it."

"The pain was there when I came out from the drugs. I became aware of the pains in the arms, underneath in the elbow and wrists. I complained so much they X-rayed it in case it was broken. It's been there since. Pain in my arms is like when you go really cold and they go numb. Then you decide to warm them up and as they come around you don't know whether to laugh or cry, a tingling numbness. It is also in the stomach and right hip and back. But they are different sorts of pains. Today it is my right ankle; maybe I have hurt it because it is weak.

"It is so bad, three days out of seven that I cannot do much. The worst thing is that you plan things and then they don't happen. It takes three hours to get going in the morning. As soon as you wake you know. I tend to sit with my arms up against my chest because it reduces the pain a little.

"Sometimes you can sleep, sometimes not. Sometimes you try to do things, sometimes you can't even try. Today is a good day—it is there but I can function. If bad, you just tend to curl up and hide. In some way you get used to it. On the other hand, physically there are so many things you can't do because of the pain. I was offered pain management, but I turned it down. My mind is pretty good and I did not feel I needed it. You just have to resist it. Possibly I am good at doing this, maybe not. I am not sure why sometimes I can do this but at others I cannot. I don't believe that the pain gets worse, so it must be in the mind.

"The reason I don't drink much is that with alcohol I may not be drunk but my legs will not work. It affects the central nervous system in an exaggerated way. I have been carried out of some great places, not because I am drunk, but because my thinking processes don't work. I've tried cannabis, but it is no use."

It must be mentally exhausting to have to keep such pain at bay. Finding drugs of no use, he turned to distractions and hobbies. He had been a keen painter before the injury and has returned to it.

"I started painting when I got out of bed, and could hardly hold the brush. I wanted to get the hand to work. I could only hold the brush for two to three minutes because I had no energy. A huge amount of mental energy was needed. Just, for example, to lift my foot up requires huge mental energy. The mental energy to get those nerves to fire up those muscles was remarkable. The pain side . . . I do it, but it takes me a long time, I have a rule, I have to be out by 10. Wherever I am, I have to be going somewhere. Just for a cup of coffee. Otherwise it would be so easy to just lie there. Now there are some mornings when I hardly get out for the pain is so bad."

The sheer amount of effort and energy needed to function in the face of weakness is difficult to describe, though it is a well-known phenomenon, perhaps best described clinically by a neuroanatomist after his stroke.[2] The chronic tiredness of having to live with pain is another thing.

Bob had been a financial consultant and had considered going back part time, but he found he just could not concentrate. It was not the loss of sensation or impoverished movement, nor his wasted body; pain prevented him from functioning.

"I always hate sympathy, but you do need some understanding. The problem is that your condition is beyond the understanding of many. My quality of life has halved, the things that I cannot do now matter so much, particularly windsurfing, running around—now I am tethered to a certain place."

Tethered seemed entirely correct; he was unable to move far or fast with his problems, and so his passage through the world had been fundamentally altered. Distances that had been trivial were now insuperable. Stairs and steep hills were beyond him. Without even a wheelchair to allow some relaxation in movement, he was tethered to a few accessible places. In the end, though, he did windsurf, once.

"Finally I did sail across to a sand bank and back. Took an hour—a minute and half on the water and the rest getting ready. My friends helped, but said they would not help again until I was stronger. It was very difficult, with my balance and strength and control."

Bob told me of his wife. "Rachel is a wonderful person. She was my PA, and I rang her up from Switzerland. I was staying in an old palace with a bimbo. The bimbo said I was snoring—in those days I was attractive to women. I thought this was ridiculous, so I got her bedding and put it in the bathroom and told her to sleep in there.

"I rang Rachel and said that I needed some stability in my life and I had decided she was it. She had the keys to my flat, so I said I'd be back in four days, move your stuff in. She said, 'Piss off. You are over there with that blond bimbo,' and put the phone down. Four weeks later, she moved in. She ran my life. I had tried the falling in love thing before, but it hadn't worked. We got together and it was great."

Bob is naturally gregarious and charming, and I could see how Rachel had fallen for him. Now he was hardly able to be sociable at all.

"That's why I spend time on my own. I do not want to inflict myself on others when I am bad. I try to avoid pain stopping me doing something. Unless it stops me completely. . . . You've got to resist. You must not feel sorry for yourself. Sometimes you want to hide, but you keep going. I have been helped by a business psychology approach, the psychology of achievement. Whatever you believe becomes your reality. Behavioral science is so important: why does one walk and the other not? Expectation. Doctors on the whole do not lay enough emphasis on this."

Toward the end of our talk he mentioned that he and Rachel would probably have split anyway. Then, rather casually, he added that once he had phoned a friend to ask him to come by because Rachel was throwing furniture out the window at his car.

Torn

Bob left to meet his daughter and, as he did, Rachel arrived. She told me that Bob had been injured nearly eight years before in the South of France, in a car crash. After the neck stabilization operation he was air ambulanced back to a spinal center.

"He was told he would not walk again—a great motivator—but one which has to be used carefully. The downside was pain. Relentless pain is the worst thing to live with. I knew from talking to him about it and seeing it etched on his face. But it is also behavioral. I went through six months when I barely slept. He was in so much pain that sharing a bed was impossible. It was just irritability, anger . . . seeing him in pain was terrible.

"When he spent months in hospital for rehab, I drove back and forth, but I got used to living on my own. He started to come home for weekends and then took his own discharge and came back here permanently. That was OK, but then it became very difficult and life changing for us all. His needs and those of our daughter were so conflicting that I was torn.

"It was also difficult having to cope with his behavior. The man who came back was different to the one I had married and had a child with. Physically he had aged and shrunk. Mood swings, irritability, pain. . . . I think we could have coped with the physical disability, I really do. We tried very hard for two to three years to make it work, but it was difficult to bring up a child.

"Initially we thought it would be better for our daughter if we were together. I also felt a lot of guilt. Might Bob be resentful if I was the one who walked away? Though there was an eighteen-year age gap, I would have coped. But I was the target of his anger and frustration.

"He had been a self-employed management consultant, having been a senior manager in a company for eighteen years after the army. He had been bringing money in, and then suddenly that stopped. This knocked his self-esteem; then he became impotent, and that created all sorts of other problems. I thought I could have dealt with it, but for him it was another thing he could not deal with, and there was a lot of anger. We just destroyed each other.

"Then there were all the other things, and the insurance and compensation claims. Trying to get benefits was a struggle for us as reasonably intelligent people, so I fear for some others. The stress levels were so high we lived a terrible time. They argued that he had some mobility so he should go to work, and he had to say it was not the movement difficulties, it was the pain that stopped him working.

"He could never commit himself because he would never know from one day to the next how he would be. On a given day, the pain might be so severe that he could not keep appointments and so he could not be employed. In the end we won. We had to get three neurologists to agree that he would never work again, and then the insurance policy paid. But to be given a diagnosis of permanent disability was a mixed blessing. Having a young wife and child he could not provide for anymore was a big blow to his ego."

To the Wall

"His whole life is controlled by his pain and its unpredictability. It is always there to some degree.

"I now have to work to provide for us. He can, however, provide some childcare and can always have our daughter during the school holidays, except when the pain is severe, and then suddenly he cannot do it. At times he just wants to turn his face to the wall. As a culture we always think we overcome pain, so when we have pain and we cannot deal with it, we come up against a wall. He paints well and was very blessed that he did not lose that skill. It is mentally absorbing and allows him to shut himself off from the pain."

I was reminded of how Renoir, toward the end of his life and in great pain, painted more and more. On the day of his death he painted anemones, forgetting his pain while he did.[3]

"Bob's quality of life is nothing compared with what it was. Sociability has suffered. He is very solitary. He has a core group that support him, but if they had not been close friends they may not have put up with him.

"He began to get violent. It was at that stage that I had to make a decision. It got worse financially. He started making purchases without my knowledge. He ran up an enormous credit card bill, buying pleasure-seeking things and going to bars and gambling, I think. Though I can now remove myself from this, and say, OK, it was a reaction, I could not sustain marriage with the lies and deceit. . . . He was forging my signature, and when confronted with it would deny and be angry. It was a combination of pain and lost mobility. But also not being able to work gave him a lot of time, empty time, which he had not had before. How could he fill his time? At that time he probably was drinking. The impotence was probably relevant there too, and him not feeling attractive to the opposite sex. Maybe that's why he was going out, trying to attract others. I was happy he was not seeing another, since I knew he could not, but maybe at the visual level he was, and he certainly appeared to be trying to see if he could attract them. He would throw money around. A ghastly time, and I had to defend my daughter from it. Credit cards bills came through, and I would see where he had spent it, and knew we could not pay.

"Sex is fundamental. . . . I was thirty, and it had been a good part of our marriage. He would not talk about it, even if there had been someone to talk about it to. I could have found a way round it, but he would not let me see him naked because he was wasted and scarred. It was not just the intercourse; it was the whole touching, kissing thing. He just felt so unattractive and turned away. Why would this young attractive wife want anything to do with him? And to me that was a rejection. I wanted to see what we could do.

"Also his skin is sensitive to touch, it was like a burning, which prevented us doing much. He was a fit man and a very attractive man. Suddenly these two things—attractive to women and a well-paid lifestyle—were denied him, and there was the pain, too.

"He had never been jealous. In fact, he quite liked other men paying me attention, knowing I was his. But after the accident that completely changed, so that every man I talked with provoked an angry reaction, even though there was no need. In a way it was almost a relief when I left. He felt he was unworthy of me. I really wanted the marriage to work, but it was not going to happen, and I had to walk away for our daughter's sake. I walked away knowing I could do no more.

"It has got better since then. We occasionally have little outbursts. I am in a new relationship now, and he has been much better since then. There is a sense that the responsibility has shifted; he had let me down and now someone else has taken it up. He knows that I will care for him, and always will, and he has a strong relationship with his daughter. Whatever, I will still support him. My new man knows this, too. Divorce is not what I want. If I am completely honest, I think it will only be a matter of time before he dies and somehow it will be better for him and for our daughter then. I would love to remarry now, but it seems not right while he is alive. I never thought he would last this long. He has had serious septicemia and lived, and should never have survived the accident. He wants to live. Sheer willpower. I respect this.

"At his worst, with the pain and seeing him crippled with it, it is just terrible to see. The loss of mobility was not so bad, but the pain has been a whole different area I had not thought of previously.

"I am never sure whether Bob feels easier with new people he meets after, or people from before, and I am not sure he knows, either. That's why he spends so much time alone. Anyone who knew him before must pity him. At least with new people they are judging for what he is now. But then he is not as attractive as he was, so he cannot bring anything, so to compensate he does not try to be happy.'"

The loss of Bob's physical presence must have been very difficult. He had been a very masculine, embodied man, proud of his time in the army, of his windsurfing, and of his physicality. His injury affected the things he held most dear and that defined him in the eyes not only of others, but also of himself.

His partial recovery may have been a mixed blessing. True, he could walk, but in the end, being neither a proper walker nor in a wheelchair may have deprived him of either a "healthy" identity or of an easily recognized impaired one; he was neither fish nor fowl. Worse, being able to walk—just—is a constant reminder of what used to be, and has prevented him from breaking with the past.

Perhaps I was just naive, but I was surprised by the differing perceptions of Bob and Rachel. Above all their stories showed some of the effects of living with the injury, the loss of mobility, and the loss of work and independence. Maybe these might all have been assimilated, but it was the chronic pain that had been so destructive to his marriage and family, work, social relationships, and self-esteem. It destroyed concentration, sociability, relationships, and income. It had eaten away, invisibly, at Bob himself. Paralysis does not stop a life, but pain may.

12 | **Both Sides Now**

Julie Hill's book *Footprints in the Snow*[1] is as much about her injury and her response as it is about her ground breaking LARSI journey (despite, one suspects, her publisher's wishes). Within her account, her husband's help and his responses to her living from a wheelchair are never far from the surface. She had discussed with him some of her thoughts during writing, but not all. Talking with Kevin, then, gave a chance to see how their perspectives and memories compared.

Julie's Kevin

Kevin, Julie suggested rightly, had not been keen on her taking a job once the children were back at school. She was desperate to find something else apart from being a mother, something else that was about her. She had been laid off from a couple of jobs before, which just made her more anxious to succeed in this. But the job as a brewery representative—power suits for lecherous landlords—was not what Kevin had wanted at all. This was one of several reasons, she suggested, for them drifting apart, even before the injury. Though they needed the money, her new independence was, she realized, a threat to him.

Julie's initial memories of Kevin after her injury are patchy—she was gravely ill and for a time, at least, out of it. She does mention how, when he and Julie got to Odstock, he sat in a corner by the desk as lots of people wheeled past in chairs. She described a "corridor full of empty wheelchairs, alien shapes reflected in polished lino. . . . Kev suddenly felt surrounded . . . physically winded. That was the moment of impact, rather than the original injury. Trembling from head to toe, blinking back the tears."

To start with he was there most of the day and night. Then, once the immediate threat was passed, he had to have some time off to attend to work and to the boys. He remembers coming back when Julie was waking. "I had been there for twenty-four hours a day for five days, and then I went for a short time. When I came back she said, 'About time you turned up.'"

Because he had just changed jobs, Kevin was reluctant to tell them at work about the accident, so he worked and then drove each night to see Julie, while juggling the needs of their children and concerns of Julie's parents. Once she was over the early acute period, and seeing him struggle, she made him tell them at work. The firm was, in fact, very understanding and flexible. When, soon after, she realized that she would not walk again, her immediate thought was that Kevin would either leave her or stay out of resentment and obligation. As the weeks turned to months, he was unable to sustain the work, the care for the family, and the visits. Something had to give, and he reduced his trips to the hospital. Julie knew he had to be mother and father all in one, but his absences were still difficult to take.

She also knew that they were both angry at the unfairness of it all, and that they raged at each other, too. She intellectualized that "Why me?" was asked as much by people close to those in wheelchairs as those in them. But still, she felt, Kevin was seeing the disability and not her. He became "paranoid about chairs, ever since that first night. Having never noticed them, he started to see them wherever he went—supermarket, street, pub, driving home. A conspiracy . . . seeing one in the middle of the day was enough to turn his blood cold. Wheelchairs swamped him by day and haunted him by night."

When it was time for Julie to try a chair herself, Kevin was "stony faced and silent, jaw clenching and unclenching as he fought to control his emotions. . . . A wheelchair represented his worst fears, a point of no return." On what was to have been his first day out with Julie in a chair,

Kevin was given instructions on how to help with Julie's transfers from chair to car and so on. He could not go through with it; her brother went with her instead.

There was an awful party for Julie's twenty-ninth birthday, when all her hospital friends and nurses stayed together at one end of the room while Kevin and his friends and colleagues were up the other. Julie wrote of her wheelchair friends putting him off and how the "disability had affected him as much as or more than her." But, she added, he "had choices that she did not." Julie thought Kevin was still seeing the chair and not her.

To have some time together, Julie had been suggesting a holiday, and finally Kevin agreed. They got away and had a ball, laughing—really laughing—together for the first time in months. But for Julie it was not for some years later, when she began the LARSI work, that she and Kevin really were together again. And, in part, this began when he finally talked of his problems. This opening up was, to an extent, because he got to know and trust the TV crew after nearly a year's filming. He talked because, rather prosaically, they asked him. It was the first time someone had actually asked him what he felt.

During the long experiments with the LARSI system, as they tried to optimize the stimulation settings, Julie was pleased to see Kevin as involved as she was. He helped not only with transport but by making suggestions himself. It was as though the LARSI had reawakened his interest in her.

By the end of her book, it is clear how much both she and Kevin had been through both separately and then together, and how they had reached a relationship and understanding of each other that is deeper now than before the injury. But never does Julie shy away from saying how trying some of their times together had been.

Kevin's Julie

It must have been difficult for Kevin to agree to meet me, because of the times I was interested in, and because I would almost be an interpreter between husband and wife. We sat in the lounge, plied with tea by Julie. He began to remember.

"I was woken by the police, and they were concerned she might not survive. The kids were four and six. I got the in-laws around and her

Dad came with me, while Mum stayed at home. We went to hospital and the doctor told us that she would not walk again. We knew then— though I did not know what it really meant. My attitudes towards wheelchairs were not favorable. I hardly noticed them up till then. . . . I thought that those in a wheelchair might have a mental problem as well.

"When we got to Odstock I sat in the corner by the desk on the wall and someone, then lots of people, came past in chairs, and at that time, I saw the impact of being in a wheelchair and what it would mean for house and home, life and everything. In the beginning it was very difficult. I am not good in hospital. Also I was not good with company, especially when, after a while, she was most comfortable with her friends in there, since they saw each other every day. We were just visiting from outside."

When Julie was ill in intensive care, it must have been awful for Kevin. But, in a curious way, when she was critically ill, needing support, prayer, and rallying around, Kevin knew what was expected. Terrible though it was, and though he had never had to deal with this before, there were rules. But then as the weeks started to pass, another period began that led them to completely new territories, territories that turned out to be very different for each of them.

Once the emergency was over, Julie's rehab, which she took to so enthusiastically and wholeheartedly, drew her into the community of the unit at the expense of her relationships with people outside, and especially at the expense of Kevin. He wanted Julie back, and shared and admired her motivation. But he had little knowledge of spinal cord injury, of chairs, of rehab, or of Julie's new needs and requirements. The new life that had been forced onto her did not overlap with his new life at all. His new life was looking after the kids and home while working full time.

Moreover, she was being supported and encouraged by a whole community of nurses, therapists, and OTs. Her new friends were patients in the same situation as her, united by one of the most dramatic events imaginable in a life. Their bonds and mutual support were huge, based on their injuries, their mutual support and encouragement, and their living together. Kevin had no entry to this, no point of reference, and little understanding or insight.

"You are left out and just pick the person up when they are sorted. There is no support for you. All friends and family are asking how is 'she,' never how you are. On reflection, had I been more agreeable with and sympathetic towards counselling then, I would have explored it. It might have been more proactive and explanatory. Two or three couples separated while Julie was in. Perhaps they might not have, had this been more available. I felt so left out of it."

Julie had the injury and a new community to help her adapt to her new situation, away from the pressures of the world. Kevin was on his own: a man of few words and with none to express his feelings and fears, and with no one to listen. Kevin adopted a routine with the boys, their school, his work, cooking, shopping, as most men would. Routine became important; so important that when Julie started going home, she disrupted it.

"When she came back for the weekend it was as though she was a visitor. I would clean the house in a certain way each time. That was very important to me; when she came back she messed up and interrupted this. It was nice to see her, but I was pleased at the end of a weekend, once she had gone. Then I could get back to the routine."

It was clear, though, that for Kevin routine was not enough, and certainly not a sufficient thing to hold onto. Julie wrote of him becoming so low that he contemplated suicide. He agreed. "It did get bad. I was feeling ostracized from Odstock. But it's one thing to contemplate taking your own life, another to do it. In the end you carry on."

This stage had been short and not serious; after all, he had a job and two boys who needed him. He continued, "At the time, and I am not sure we have discussed this, she thought the problem was with my seeing the disability and not her as a person. It was not. It was because all her friends and her new life were in the hospital and in the unit, and I could not be part of that. It was more that I was ostracized because of her rehabilitation and her being in there learning a new way. This has never really been discussed. When the book came out, I said that the editor was a man hater. The other side is never shown.

"Emotions were very difficult at that time. I had a fear of failing to cope with the various parts. Once she had a bladder blockage, and we got back into hospital faster than the doctor. Bladder and bowels are not usually part of the normal parts of one's life. She had lived with these (and been taught about them) for months before she came home. We had to get used to it together as well. I had to understand what she had learned and how she wanted me to do things. Julie had to learn to ask for help, just as I had to learn when and how to give it. She had a seven-month start, and had had months of medical humor about it all which I did not have. I can understand it now, but at the time it was difficult."

Julie had written that Kevin was, for a while, paranoid about wheelchairs, that they were a symbol of her new needs and status in a way that had more to do with his prejudice and lack of knowledge than about their use and ease. He agreed.

"It's like buying a new car and seeing everyone has one. It was a nightmare—wheelchairs were everywhere. It was a misconception, it was a ball and chain syndrome, having to look after someone, the mental loss as well, someone damaged, dribbling in the chair. It was a Dickensian attitude I had at the time. Someone dependent and with no chance of having a life with them. I knew that Julie was fine mentally . . . but I still had this thought, this wrong idea, that physical disability and a mental one go together. I think very differently now. You need to work one to one, every day joking and talking.

"Her perception was that it was me not seeing her in the chair. In fact, in my mind, it was her relationship with the hospital, and the people there, which was distancing her from me and a life outside. Her twenty-ninth birthday was a disaster. There was family, and there were those with spinal cord injury and the nurses. They had got themselves into a tight-knit community. We were not a part of it, and the groups were at opposite ends of the room all night.

"Back at home was similar. Once she got over the 'visitor syndrome at home,' it was not because of the chair and me seeing that. It was her, and her still feeling in—and not really leaving—the new community she had found. This is not to put down those at the hospital or her new friends—both are smashing. But put them together, and they were cracking jokes that you did not understand."

To an extent she had to leave her new community for this to happen. It must have been difficult, because initially she was at a very low ebb herself. She needed all the help she could get to gain a sense of her self as valid and useful. This was part of what Odstock was helping her with. It was just that this identity depended on, and was immersed in, a coming to terms with and acceptance of her impairment. The need was to absorb this sufficiently that she could then be outward looking again, saying,

"Yes I am paraplegic, but am I more than that." The first step was, inevitably, inward. Was she a paraplegic, or a person with paraplegia? What was her identity with and without the spinal cord injury, and how did they co-exist? These were balances no one could really help her with, or even discuss. One might accept being paraplegic and, rightly, proud of one's living with it, but still be aware that this might distance one from others. Kevin agreed. "She was more at one with her new community and had to leave that."

Leaving was made easier by a weekend in a bungalow attached to the hospital, where they were independent and left alone. But Kevin suggested it was sometime after she had left that gradually they got back to talk to each other each night. I was reminded of the parallel experiences of a friend, James Partridge, who had suffered severe burns to the face and body. He had had surgery for several years and been left with some residual facial difference, making him the object of staring in most public places. He had received wonderful surgical and medical support, but no psychosocial education. When discharged from the hospital, he had no idea how to look someone in the eye, or any idea how to initiate a conversation, or order a pint of beer. It took James seven years of trial and error to learn these social skills.[2] Julie had received rehabilitation in the necessary bowel and bladder care, in pressure area vigilance and in transfers, but no advice in how to take up her life anew with others, or how to diffuse and reduce the problems of distancing between her, as a paraplegic, and other able-bodied people, and especially between her and her husband.

Kevin thinks this should be addressed. "It can be awkward if people are left out, whether families or their new friends. They actually need in spinal units to give patients help in relearning social skills, one on one, for when they leave." He added that they will also need, of course, to keep up with their new friends from their new world. "There need to be two programs, one for the one who's injured, to learn about the outside world again, and then one for the families to understand the new circumstances of the injured person."

"Our first holiday in Rhodes was good. They said there were facilities for disabled people, but we did not want to use them, so where we went there were steps. One couple got us some lounge chairs every day, and the man was always there to help lift over the steps. They would drag the lounge out of the sun to prevent Julie getting sunburned. Their over-concern helped us get our sense of humor back. We laughed with it and against it and as one. Humor worked by stealth in the end."

All this had happened a little while after Julie had been discharged. I moved onto the documentary and when Kevin had finally talked of his feelings.

"No one had asked me before. The film crew had been around for over twelve months, and we had a good rapport, and it just came out. Previously I had bottled up my emotions and just got on with the routine. I did grieve for what I had lost very early on, in my own confines. . . . Not when she was initially ill, but once the operation was over and the transition began. No one knew at the time. Friends would rally around Julie and go to see her, but no one came around for me. You start to reflect after a while. But you don't go looking for support—I had my routine and that was it.

"For one or two months I was depressed and grieving, but never since—that becomes self-indulgent. We have had our moments trying to find each other again. Living together under one roof was important."

LARSI

In Julie's book, Kevin was a very enthusiastic supporter of the LARSI system. More than that, at times his common sense and practicality led to genuine advances in the technology. He had seen her somewhat misplaced, though understandable, enthusiasm for at least one other mobility aid lead to weeks of effort followed by disappointment. By the time the call for LARSI volunteers arrived, he had adapted to her new life in a chair.

"I had this viewpoint, why did she want to do it? Because it does not matter if she does not walk again. Why go through all the pain and bother? Then she explained the benefits for her legs and heart and for her bones later in life. Forget walking, I thought, these were sufficient. Then, if she could stand, great. No one ever mentioned walking. As she built up her muscles with the functional electrical stimulation, over the months I could see her well-being improving.

"The whole purpose of the muscle build up was the LARSI, but she needed her bone and muscles built up anyway. I could see, even before the operation, a definite benefit. Suddenly there was logic behind this and we could discuss it together. I could see she would do it and go forward.

"We met the people and they were smashing. Then, when it happened, I could actually make a contribution . . . and it was nice that they were willing to listen. I came up with an idea for the chair and got some plates made. They were all too intelligent sometimes and impractical. They also had a good rapport with no hierarchies. There were jokes, too. They occasionally thought it was not working and would turn it all off and she would collapse like potatoes."

Kevin was animated and describing this as a joint experiment, something they both were able to partake in. Given his enthusiasm and practical skills, I wondered if he could have helped earlier, when she was learning to transfer and get into a wheelchair?

"I can only give a hypothetical answer. The way my emotions were running at the time it would have been a struggle to do that. But perhaps the right person in the right manner saying the rights things might have persuaded me. But even then the timing was wrong. Later with the research I could see it doing her good.

"I was totally caught up in the LARSI. I could see the benefits for her, and then, when I got involved with the team—another community—who were such a smashing bunch, with a sense of humor, it clicked. OK, I got frustrated at times—we wanted to take it home at one point and they said no. It ended up as a joke between the two of us. It was the first time we had discussed things directly to do with her disability."

Once the LARSI had been implanted with an external control box it was possible for Kevin to share the stimulation. Then, with shared control he had some involvement and a shared sense of ownership of her movement. This was what initially had brought them together once more.

"I was helping the doctors in where they were going. I could get captured by it. The only problem was in a way when it was finished. It was OK when the TV program came out and we went to various places, but then suddenly everyone had moved on and we were left. You had got used to enjoying it. It was not so much these fringe benefits. It was the team around us for fourteen months and then gone. No filming. . . . You wonder what they are doing. . . . It is like losing friends."

Now that the LARSI project has faltered, Kevin can look back more impassively.

"There was the standing, which was the goal, and then the possibility of walking, and then we were deflected into cycling. The trike worked, but Julie finds it difficult and it does not happen much. It is the 'faff factor' for her, 'Do I really want to do it?' Because she always needs someone to help her into it, it is not something she can do on her own, and so does not allow her true independence.

"We did all want it to work so much, and it nearly did. But even without the walking we have standing and the trike, more than we expected. Frustrating, yes, but never a disappointment. We have done lots and seen lots. I would never decry them for trying, nor the result we have."

I wondered if Julie might be more disappointed, due to the instability when standing?

"This might come from them being deflected onto the trike and away from stepping. The one time we thought it might be nice to have crutches to allow her to step and 'walk' around the house, but we did not get there. The trike is not independence, so that it technically is a step back, though I would not knock them for that.

"At times they were too intelligent. Occasionally you wanted them to play with it and use trial and error. They could get so involved in the data. We argued, though the rapport was good. We got a lot more than we expected."

In retrospect, problems first arose around the time of rehabilitation and then around the trial periods at home, problems both Julie and Kevin saw, but from very different viewpoints. For Julie to integrate her new identity as paraplegic with her continuing roles as mother and wife could not have been easy. She needed the support and sense of community available to her in the hospital. This culture and camaraderie was essential, though they kept her from Kevin.

She saw him looking at the chair; he saw her with her new disabled identity and culture, distancing her from his everyday life. An obvious way of avoiding this is to include families and husbands and wives in the rehabilitation programs at an early stage. Yet Kevin was reluctant to endorse this. Early on he was so ambivalent about the hospital and wheelchairs and spinal injury that it might have been too big a thing to contemplate and might have been counterproductive. In the end, his old phobias about wheelchairs disappeared, and now he seeks out people in chairs to talk to. If there was a way to bring people into the experiences of their loved ones, learning of their new lives, then this might reduce the early divorces and separations that may occur after spinal cord injury.

Nigel North actually tried to start a program at Odstock for the wives and husbands of patients, but it was not taken up by sufficient numbers to make it worthwhile. Perhaps it is too early after the event for people to come to terms with it and learn about the practicalities.

For Kevin, the LARSI has been a huge success, not solely for the scientific advances or for the motivation it gave Julie, or even for giving her choices in standing or cycling. Its success for him was also in enabling him to take part as an equal in an aspect of Julie's care. "It was the first time we had discussed things directly to do with her disability."

People with physical impairments need to manage their own problems in their daily lives as best they can. Although there is still controversy as to whether they should be defined by their impairment or disability, or be defined like anyone else by their achievements and failures, loves and losses, it seems less controversial that they must go beyond their disabled identities to find ways of sharing their lives with their loved ones. Equally important, their loved ones have to find ways to share the new, altered, lives of their partner. The LARSI project gave Kevin and Julie a shared language and a shared life once more.

As Kevin related, one of the most distressing things about Julie's injury was that it distanced him from her. This, in part, was a consequence of the self-centeredness that was so necessary for Julie during her early rehabilitation. Something similar was described in another context by Matt Seaton, the partner of a woman dying of cancer: "I often felt, as Ruth was dying, our relationship was by degrees dying with her. . . . I just wish—how I wish—that I could have somehow got round it: loved Ruth or made her feel loved, in the old way, to the very end. But cancer changed everything: it put us on different tracks, stretching our grasp of one another to the limit and eventually forcing us apart."[3]

Somehow people have to find ways of reducing the gap between the injured and themselves, to see each side's perspective and to continue to share their lives as those lives themselves change. This section was called

"Observing," but in truth the family and friends of someone newly injured do far more than observe.

We now move to the stories of two tetraplegic men who have coped with their impairment with great outward success. More than this, however, both have gone on to become active in the disability movement and been influential in improving the social provisions for people with spinal cord injury and disability in general. In doing so, they have both questioned the concepts underlying the very notion of disability and challenged doctors and politicians alike to redefine their terms and their practices.

VI

Empowering

Disability Matters

Medicine by Default

Stephen's parents had just qualified in medicine, in Liverpool, when he was born. Soon they moved to London to practice, but after a short time in "the smoke," moved to the more genteel parts of Surrey and Sussex, around Crawley and then Epsom. Stephen was educated at a private prep school, then at Epsom College, a medical foundation school that "churned out medics." He describes becoming a doctor almost by default, as a result of a "genetic impairment" (medicine certainly used to run in families, like alcoholism and teenage pregnancies). His elder brother went to medical school in Southampton, and Stephen ended up at Guys in London. By then his mother was in family planning, and his father was professor of oral medicine at the Royal London Hospital. His sister, Stephen said tactfully, did not make the grade academically and so became a nurse.

As a boy he loved sailing and rugby. At school, except when exams were close, he got by without too much effort. He didn't work hard and didn't need to. He managed the grades for medical school without much problem and, once there, threw himself into the social scene, with rugby and sailing to the fore again.

The course was a traditional one, so for the first two years he covered the basic sciences. It was like school, only (slightly) more grown up.

Then for the third year, he graduated to clinical study and began seeing real live patients, and what was more, patients from inner city London. Immediately he felt awkward and even, at times, embarrassed. He found it difficult to talk to ordinary people—after all, he had never had to before. Suddenly he became aware of a cultural mismatch between who he was and who they were, local people from Bermondsey. He found a way of avoiding talking with patients as people, zeroing in on medical symptoms and signs—his newfound medical jargon and a white coat a carapace.

It was at the end of his third year at medical school in the early 1980s, during a surgical rotation with Professor McColl, that he went with some friends for rugby training. He had been captain of the Second XV the year before and had played for the First team too, so he was well known within the sport.

"Twenty-first of September, 7 p.m., during a preseason training session, I did a crash tackle, fell, and broke my neck. I lay there for a couple of hours without losing consciousness, though I phased in and out a bit. It was a very hot day, but I remember it going dark and cold. The ambulance took three hours coming from Kings, one and a half miles down the road. They had a message I had broken my leg rather than my neck. I was admitted to Kings for forty-eight hours, and then I was moved by ambulance to Stoke Mandeville.

"I knew straight away. Lots of rugby player friends had told me, 'If you play like that, one day you will break your neck.' Also there had been a boy at school, two years older than me, who broke his neck playing rugby.

"I couldn't feel anything from my neck down, apart from pain.

"The first few bits were quite challenging. While in hospital at Kings they wouldn't give me any analgesia or anesthetic because my blood pressure was so low and they were worried about my breathing and things. So they put in the halo brace without anesthetic, drilling holes in my head with me being worried they would go too far and hit my brain. I was intubated, so I couldn't even talk."

Once stabilized, he was taken to Stoke Mandeville. His professor came to see him, spending two hours with Stephen, and his mother and father. As he left, he said something Stephen has never forgotten: "Don't worry, you will qualify as a doctor."

"I knew then whatever happened that it was OK. All my student life was sorted. All those worries had been taken away. Not that I suppose I ever really wanted to be a doctor, but it was reassuring."

In relating his story with exuberance and humor, Stephen suddenly stopped and realized he had missed out the most important thing about his pre-accident experience—he had fallen desperately in love with Rose. They had been living together for about eighteen months; he had proposed six weeks before the accident, and she had agreed to marry him.

"When she came to see me, I was intubated with a tube down my throat. I started blinking because I thought I can't move my arm, my head, I can't talk—I need to communicate. I was on a Stryker frame, where they tip you [to avoid pressure sores to any given area]. I could not feel my body and thought I was being turned head over heels even though I was being rotated in an axial plane, I think.

"She sussed eventually that one blink was yes and two was no. It took two hours to sort that out, with me crying and her pleading as she tried to work out what was going on. Then she drew an alphabet and we did yes, yes, yes, no, no, no, as we got to the right letter and I could spell words out."

Fortunately the tube was not in for long.

Hell's Angels and Pantomime Horses

His uncle, a neurologist, came over from the States with support and help.

"He placated Mum and Dad—well, not placated them, told them the worst, really. That was quite important.

"Then because my pulse and blood pressure were so low, they bunged some atropine in and I went completely loopy. I think there were two reasons why I went mad. First of all, the side-effect of the drug, and secondly I was getting some sensory recovery. My hallucinations lasted for about forty-eight to seventy-two hours, and were based around me being tortured. I was attacked by a bunch of Hell's Angels, and they were lacerating my skin every half centimeter and injecting petrol and setting fire to it. I imagine it was something to do with the sensory loss and it coming back partially, and the way my brain was suddenly deprived of so much and decided to make stuff up. It was a fascinating experience.

"Another hallucination was of my bowels being pulled inside out, some-one reaching inside me physically, from my mouth, and disconnecting my intestines and pulling them out so they were flowing behind me."

He was not sure if the feeling of hovering at this time, as though in mid space, was a hallucination or was the correct feeling, because he could feel nothing below the neck. Whatever, it intensified the terror.

Stephen came really alive as he told me all this, with a wonderful boy-ish enthusiasm. He had tried to tell people at the time, but they had not believed him.

"I had them all cowering down behind the bed to keep out the way, and my Mum and Dad said how stupid they felt hiding because I was screaming. 'Hide, hide!' at the top of my voice. I had pantomime horses with blood dripping off their savage metallic teeth, climbing over me and eating me."

They stopped the atropine.

"I was a complete pain on the ward because I was screaming all the time and the other patients were trying to sleep. Time in hospital wasn't good. I had no movement in either arm for most of the time. Then I started to get some flickers of movement in my thumb to begin with, and in biceps.

"They sat me up later than usual, at around sixteen weeks, because my neck fracture was a bit unstable—it's usually twelve weeks, I think. Sitting was weird. I had started to get the sensation back. Other patients were saying it's a bit like having a ghost's head. You are wandering around but cannot feel your body. By then I had some feeling in my body, so I didn't go through that, but I was very spastic to begin with, so I was stiff and had spasms which set me back. But after that I made friends with the other patients and we just had fun. We had been dealt our fate and we were getting on with it."

I was amazed he could have fun, but he insisted he did. One guy, nicknamed Snoopy, was a sixteen-year-old paraplegic boy. They got him drunk at the pub one day and he came back vomiting all over the ward. He fell out of bed a couple of times. He was banned from going out of the ward for a week, so the others waited until the staff were busy with a changeover, tied his bed to an electric wheelchair and towed him to the local staff club. They were on their second pint before they were found.[1]

Stephen's return of sensation occurred within a few weeks. He was left with a complete motor injury at C3/C4 but, surprisingly, with some finger movement in the right hand, with sparing of sensation there, so that he can feel light touch and vibration. This one hand is his lifeline and allows him considerably more useful movement than someone with a severe cord injury at this level can normally expect. His sensation meant that he was fortunate to feel his first bowel motion after the accident and have a warning. His bladder and bowel care was taught and accepted as "just something that was done."

During his time in the hospital his neurologist uncle sent him a tape every month about some neurological condition. His father rigged up a television by his bed on a tripod on wheels. He also had a video player and so could watch videos about pathology and other medical matters. In the days long before hospital TVs, these helped keep his mind active and reduced the boredom and introspection.

Because of the high level of his injury in the neck there was not a huge amount of physiotherapy possible. After nine months, he was discharged.

Wheelchair Student

He went back home to his parents for three months of recuperation before returning to Guys again in the September. An occupational therapist had managed to commandeer a council flat within wheelchair distance of Guys, and it was fixed up with a hoist in the ceiling, ramped access, and a door Stephen could operate. Rose became, just into her twenties, sole carer. A physiotherapy student, she had taken a year out to help at Stoke Mandeville. This was all despite the fact that Stephen had told her, in the first week, that he didn't want to see her again.

"I didn't think it was fair on her. I told her to go away. I didn't want her to see me with all this stuff happening."

She refused to go. She hung in, and Stephen hopes that she is pleased that she did. But for two years, they had a difficult time. To be a sexual partner, lover, and carer all in one must have been at times near impossible, especially for one so young. Fortunately they managed to find some support for a carer from an unlikely source. *Crossroads* was a much-loved TV soap based on a fictional motel (at a time when Britain did not really have motels). Its popularity, to a large degree, was due to its being underfinanced, so that the actors and the sets were pretty creaky. Then one actor developed multiple sclerosis in real life. Rather than write him out, they had him feign a spinal cord injury, because that was considered more socially acceptable. Then someone wrote to the producer of the program saying they had not portrayed it accurately. This goaded them into giving some funds for care, and the "Crossroads Care Attendance Scheme" was born. It allowed Rose some precious time off.

Stephen seemed set up in his flat, close to Guys and with Rose and some external support. But then his parents arrived one day with an architectural plan of the ground floor of their home with a little bit added for him, like a granny annex. They presented it with pride as a surprise, and almost as a fait accompli.

"They only did it because they loved and cared for me, not for any other reason. 'We are going to build this and you can live here.' I always say in seminars, 'What would have happened if I'd let them go ahead and build it, where would I be right now? I would be there and that generosity and kindness would have trapped me into a situation of dependency.' Rose and I said we are not doing that. There was a bit of a family argument about it."

Stephen liked understatement.

He went back to medical school, against much resistance. His father was on the General Dental Council at the time and he was talking with the General Medical Council. He was told not to make an issue of it, but to have Stephen quietly work his way back in. Unfortunately, the University of London would not accept him, so he took the alternative, but equally valid, route of taking the older examinations of the Royal Colleges of Surgery and Medicine. Being back at Guys was fine; they did not mind him, even if the university did. He did his pathology finals with his original year because the Dean had said they wanted to check if his brain was still in order. He passed and was back on the course.

"I was wearing a white coat, I had a stethoscope around my neck and I was whizzing around in a wheelchair when I should have been a patient."

But much more than his mode of getting around the wards had changed. His ability to talk with patients had been completely turned around.

"You know I mentioned before about how incompetent I felt at interacting with other patients. I felt brilliant at doing it by then. In fact, I was so proud of how I had changed as a person, the significant advantage I got out of the experience. I could spend hours talking to people who were dying. Before I would never have gone there, it was too scary.

"I'd been a patient. I understood how important it is for someone to spend time with you. I remember times when my consultant at Stoke would come along and say, 'Pull your toes up,' to see if I was getting any further recovery. I'd be straining away doing it, and Rose would be by my side because she used to come in for the ward round, and the consultant would be three patients down by then, and I wouldn't have had any feedback or any conversation."

It is difficult to underestimate this change. In the 1980s medical students were not renowned for their sensitivity, especially the rugby playing hearties. Sympathy for patients was not then high up on anyone's list of desirable qualities in a doctor. Knowledge of the causes and treatment of disease was essentially all that the course required.[2]

The Time of Pus

It was a year after his return to Guys, two years after the injury, when he noticed a small blemish on the inside of his leg. Professor McColl saw him at home and decided to excise it. He operated on Stephen, there and then in his own home. Unfortunately, this did not work and soon pus started coming from the hole in his leg. He had to be admitted to the hospital. Stephen chose Guys rather than Stoke Mandeville. He spent the next five months on his back, "pouring pus."

They would get him up to make him sit, and he would pass out. At one stage they had the psychologists in because they thought the temperatures Stephen was spiking were psychogenic. They finally X-rayed his hip and found that it was shot to pieces by an infection of the bone, osteomyelitis. An orthopedic surgeon operated to open it and remove the dead bone—without an anesthetic. Stephen described this as being "quite interesting." He was given some Valium, but was still aware. They chopped away at the bone for four hours, with Stephen's head being jolted by the banging and sawing in his hip below. He smelled his flesh burning as they coagulated bleeding points. The surgeons chatted away in their jocular manner. He was scared shitless.

He was too ill to consider a claim for negligence. Eventually his physician from Stoke Mandeville was informed and came down immediately. He was absolutely furious with Guys, and with Stephen. He moved him to Stoke straight away and admitted him to intensive care. Though not in pain, Stephen had lost a huge amount of weight as the infection consumed his bone and his flesh.

A further operation by a hip specialist followed, leaving him with an even larger draining hole.

I asked why he had been so keen to avoid Stoke Mandeville.

"I had shut that door behind me; it was finished. I had done it. It was a harsh regime there with no psychological support. Whatever had gone on there, all my suffering and pain, and the humiliations of my personal needs, I had gone through. The door was closed; I was not going back."[3]

At one stage they feared that the femoral artery might be involved and decided it was inoperable. He was told that this was it, that he would "rot and die." Stephen was a little concerned by this, not least because the man opposite had rotted and died in front of him, of a complication associated with his spinal injury. But by then he was so ill that he didn't really care. For the first time, if he could have committed suicide he would have. He even asked Rose to give him pills, but she wouldn't.

Several months later, he was still very ill systemically, bone being notoriously difficult to clear of infection. Told he would either get better or die, he was discharged to his fate. Not happy about dying, Stephen went to his GP to ask for a second opinion. His father had also done some investigating, and been recommended an orthopedic surgeon at the Royal National Orthopaedic Hospital at Stanmore in North London.

Ian Bayley agreed to see him and admitted him to a special infection ward. He was prepared for another operation (one of twelve or so overall), a fourteen-hour special that at one stage involved a team of eight surgeons.

"It was osteomyelitis gone rampant. As I went into the operation, the surgeon told Rose and I that I had a 50 percent chance of dying on the table, and a good chance that if I survived they would have to do a hind quarter resection which would have led to quite some difficulties being propped up in a chair on one buttock.

"I remember coming around from the operation. The thing I remember most, and I still have to this day, is a passion for tomato soup. My first meal was tomato soup and toast. If I think happiness, I can smell tomato soup. It was like I was alive, and that was good. I haven't looked back since. I have had a couple of minor little flare-ups. Several months later my surgeon found a dressing in there, down by my knee, that had been in for a while. The whole leg was a mess, which is why one leg is a bit shorter than the other and I sit a bit skewed, but it's not a problem."

Then it was back to medical school, this time a year further down. He used other students to examine patients and told them what to look for. The most important part of any examination, however, is the history, listening to the patients describe their problems in a manner that often leads you to the diagnosis. Stephen found this part much easier now. He used a Dictaphone and had someone transcribe. He did his exams with a fellow student too, telling the student what to write. By now he had some celebrity and volunteers were easy to find. Then it was house jobs, at that time an amazingly arduous rite of passage for any young doctor. He was never going to be able to do all the night work and physical slog required, so his consultant arranged for him to do it over two years instead of one.

The Activist

Before starting this, Stephen heard of a Master's Degree in Rehabilitation Studies in Southampton. Realizing the problems in becoming a doctor, he decided to aim for that rather than to do the two years at Guys. There were six months to wait, so he asked his local GP for some ideas about what to do. He suggested going to the local Day Center. It was the first time Stephen had come across other disabled people, except for those in Stoke Mandeville.

It was revelatory.

"My eyes were opened. So this is what society does to disabled people, I thought. I started to realize the indignity of the way society treats disabled people. That was my first awakening to the exclusion. Despite my disability, I had been very privileged. My parents had bought a wheelchair-accessible vehicle and a wheelchair. There wasn't a problem; it was all sorted. Here were people who lived close by in Southwark having a hard time. Society responded to disabled people by excluding them. Go to a Day Center for disabled people and don't expect to go to university, don't expect to get a job, don't have high expectations, and certainly have low self-esteem. They had segregated transport so they went on the dial-a-ride bus instead of public transport. These were people with cerebral palsy, juvenile onset rheumatoid arthritis, mental health problems, difficulties with sight, a whole mixture grouped together by their exclusion from the mainstream."

While there he met somebody who helped him to raise funds for the MSc course, because he wanted to fund it himself. Livery Companies and the Worshipful Company of Barber Surgeons stumped up some. The Rugby Club organized a match between medical internationals and a nonmedical international XV and raised £35,000. He had promised the people who raised the money that he would put it toward a house, since moving to Southampton meant he needed a house close to the hospital. The hospital was selling its nurses' accommodation, one of the periodic madnesses of the time. He and Rose benefited. She had also qualified as a therapist and so managed to support them. Stephen was still keen to have some independence and so managed another grant from the Worshipful Company of Goldsmiths, Leathersellers, and Drapers.

In Southampton at that time, some important things were happening in the field of disability studies. First it had introduced a Care Attendance Scheme for disabled people to have support at home, forced through by two of the rehabilitation doctors, Lindsay McClellan and Ted Cantrell. Stephen had help every morning to get out of bed and two nights a week to put him back.

The MSc course enveloped and fascinated Stephen. There were people from all over the world—three from New Zealand, a couple from Hong Kong, one from Africa. Most were women, though one man was gay and introduced Stephen to equality issues. Stephen began to see parallels between the experiences of women, blacks, and the disabled. They moved from rehabilitation to politics and then to the politics of disability. The Care Attendants Scheme gave him some independence for the first time in years, and he soon found his way to the Southampton Centre for Independent Living, where he met Simon Brissendon, who had a Ph.D. in Politics and Philosophy and was president of the Student Union, as well as being a wheelchair user. Before long the two of them were driving the Centre for Independent Living forward.[4]

His course was mostly taught, but there was a thesis as well. Convinced from his own experience that medical education influenced the way disabled people were treated by doctors, his was entitled, "The Impact of Medical Education on the Attitudes of Medical Students Towards Disabled People."

He found an attitude study from the States with a check box, and tested cohorts of first year and final year medical students. He also asked for their career aspirations. He found a significant deterioration in the expressed attitude to disabled people as students went through their course, and in particular in those who wanted to be orthopedic surgeons. Much to his delight, the study had confirmed both of his prejudices. Students may come into medicine wishing to make a difference and to care, but somewhere along the way this humanity is overwhelmed by the demands of the course. Slowly, one hopes, it reemerges with experience (even in orthopedic surgeons).

Down Under

While still a medical student, Stephen, through his uncle, had managed to attend a meeting of the American Society for Handicapped Physicians. There were blind doctors, deaf doctors, doctors with all sorts of progressive disabilities, and one British medical student with tetraplegia. They gave him confidence to complete his studies, but also opened his eyes to aspects of health care beyond the medical.

Then, as he was doing the MSc, he had the opportunity to go to Australia for three months. Ian Bayley arranged for a bacteriologist to give him a trunk full of antibiotics and instructions on when to take them. He had one month each in Sydney and Melbourne, talking with community-based projects led by disabled people. They had a concept called CBR, Community Based Rehabilitation, with the assumption that true rehab could not be done in the hospital. After his experiences in England, Stephen was amazed to see disabled people running their own rehabilitation programs and, more than that, some disabled people selling their expertise to councils and running rehab for others. He came back fired with enthusiasm, determined to do a similar thing in the United Kingdom.

Typically, in talking of this, Stephen had completely omitted to tell me quite how he, able to move one arm—just—had managed to get to

Australia and back. He dismissed this; he flew initially to Singapore and rested there to avoid a long trip and its possibility of pressure sores. He learned that he could use this need for stops to his advantage and, on the way back, stopped over in Hawaii for a short holiday. In Australia, he hired a van and traveled around in the back of that, using two planks to wheel up into it. They met three friends from the MSc course in New Zealand and spent Christmas there, on the beach. Hard sand, I presumed.

It was at the stopover in San Francisco that his luck ran out. As they flew in late, they were told they would not make their connection to Britain. After a mad scramble, they saw their plane just backing off its gate to take off. They banged on the window, and it stopped to let them on. But Stephen's electric wheelchair did not make it, so from Heathrow to his parents' home, the last hundred miles or so of an amazing trip, he was folded into the back of his parents' car. The chair turned up the next day, no doubt with stories of its own.

Before he went he had arranged to research for a doctorate in disability studies. His trip had confirmed him in this, but also made him realize that he could not just be academic in his approach. He had turned, in a few years, from an unthinking Guys' rugby enthusiast to a political intellectual and disability activist. From there, however, he had gone on again, and this eventually caused him to distance himself from the growing disability movement. While a student he had begun to run disability awareness seminars, and had built up quite a network of people who had been to these and been impressed by his work. He wanted to follow these through formally.

He began his Ph.D., "Disability and Equality in Employment: The Imperative of an Integrated Approach," in 1989. It took six years. His initial idea was to assess whether disability awareness training had any effect. He wanted to show whether it produced a cultural or organizational change sufficient to alter the degree to which companies promoted recruitment and retention of either disabled staff or those who become disabled. He showed that it was only if senior executives were committed to the idea, and if there was a sufficient budget to make the necessary changes and to train all staff, that anything lasting happened. None of it worked in isolation; it needed a change in the environment, which had to be backed up by legislation.

Given his energy and enthusiasm, six years might seem a long time for a doctorate in the United Kingdom. But at the same time as embarking on this, Stephen also started on another road.

Disability Matters Limited

In parallel with working on his thesis, he had begun to work his ideas on disability awareness out in practice by giving seminars. Increasingly people asked him to do it for their company; and he realized he could make money from it. Having seen the developments in Australia, he had thought he could start providing rehabilitation services commercially. He wanted the Southampton Centre for Independent Living to morph into such a professional provider. But this idea turned out to be as big a jump in perception as his own from "rugger-bugger" to disability terrorist. He had no credibility with the local government organizations that controlled the budget and so was turned down. Nor could he convince his colleagues in the Centre for Independent Living. They wanted to continue as activists and found the leap to being paid to provide a service too much. To those in the Southampton Centre, making profit from disabled services was anathema. To Stephen, it was common sense—both advanced his cause and allowed him to support himself and Rose.

"I realized that chaining yourself to a railing achieves a certain amount, but actually getting inside organizations to bring about change is firstly warmer, secondly you can earn more, and thirdly you actually got more change."

With Simon Brissenden, who had a muscular problem and lived in a wheelchair, Stephen set up Disability Matters Limited (DML). The company concerned itself with all aspects of disability but focussed, initially at least, on awareness of the problem with employers. It started in Stephen and Rose's front room, at about the same time as he began his Ph.D. Unfortunately and unexpectedly, Simon died a few months later, and Rose ended up buying his shares in DML from his estate.[5]

Stephen threw himself into his thesis and into the business. The talks were over one or two days where he would discuss the phases of the awareness of disability by others. Most people found disability an unknown and anxious area. He would discuss how in breaking down that unease there was a first "cathartic" stage, in which people would download their anxieties, concerns, and apprehensions about disability. Then Stephen would introduce some of the advantages that those with disabilities could bring to an organization, "the truth" of how disabled people are good problem solvers because they experience so many problems in their own lives. They are often good at managing change because they manage it in their own life all the time. Then he would ask what companies were doing about disability issues in employment, access, and general provision. He ended by offering practical assistance, for instance in contacting the local disabled school to arrange interviews with potential interviewees. This was not an altruistic and general introduction; once Stephen was through the door, he wanted change and commitment.

He soon found that he could not cope with the demand for seminars. After two years of hard work at the thesis and at DML, they moved from Southampton to the countryside, living in a house at the top of a hill in a small village. As the children arrived (they now have four boys aged five to ten, who do play rugby), and as the business increased, they moved Stephen's office to the house and then started adding rooms. In the end, he moved DML to a series of buildings on a farm outside Stockbridge.

High Ups

In building up DML he did not neglect his thesis, nor wait for his thesis examination and then try to publish a few peer-reviewed papers. Someone from the Department of Employment had been to a seminar and proved handy in arranging access for Stephen to the National Advisory Council for People with Disabilities and, from there, he managed to extend his reach to the very corridors of power. As he finished his thesis, he posted it off as chapters to the then minister for disabled people, Nicholas Scott.[6]

"This guy quoted huge bits of my unfinished Ph.D. in House of Commons. When he was made minister for the disabled, I had dinner with William Hague at the Dorchester, and shortly after he introduced a bill in Parliament to promote disabled issues, the Disability Discrimination Act (DDA). Obviously lots of others were lobbying too, but I felt I had some input."

In fact, there is another reason for suggesting that his input was far from insignificant. The previous minister had been the young John Major. Stephen's first mentor, Ian McColl, had been given a peerage as Thatcher's spokesperson in the House of Lords and remained influential with Major, too. Stephen assumed this inside track might have been the reason for his being awarded an OBE soon afterwards. Though naturally dismissive of his role, Stephen's work was certainly important. I had to wonder, though, how he managed to convince the Conservatives of Thatcher's era to focus on disabled people.

"Partly by the way I look and partly because of my qualifications, they are prepared to listen. You have to understand too where they are coming from. The Conservative Party wants to decrease the money spent on benefits. How to do that? Get people off incapacity benefit. How to do that? Anti-discriminatory employment legislation so nasty employers cannot avoid giving them a job. They had not thought of it like that. So you may believe in social justice, but if you know the arguments and the audience, you can play devil's advocate and get people to think that this is the way to go."

Others have told me that they are lost at a disability meeting if on the same platform as Stephen. His visible physical problem and sheer authority take over, even before he starts to talk. One cannot understate the importance of having an eloquent protagonist for the disabled who himself is disabled when confronting and cajoling people for change.

"I appealed to their wallets. Thatcher massaged unemployment figures and put them on incapacity benefit instead. Now we have 2.1 million people on that, the result of a politically motivated act. I have never been party political, but I did learn how to appeal to them."

Another key player at this time was an organization called the Employers' Forum in Disability, where a Canadian, Susan Scott-Parker, was doing a similar thing. The EFD was rather top down and needed the credibility and practical experience that Stephen provided, just as he needed Susan and the EFD for contacts and a platform for his ideas.

By now increasingly in a world of the high ups, Stephen realized that he could have been sucked in and used as a token disabled person, with lip service paid to his ideas but no real change being made underneath. However, through his persistence and tenacity he turned this on its head.

He actually found that he was listened to more the higher in an organization he could reach. He learned to be compliant with the juniors and gatekeepers to the high and mighty and then, once established, to become more forthright. Recently he worked with Maria Eagle when she was a labour minister for the disabled. She asked him to run a day's seminar on disability awareness for her team. Stephen said he would only do it if she came too. She did.

In his basic seminars to employers and government he would deal with why there were so many people on incapacity benefit, using Elisabeth Kubler-Ross's framework for the way people react to severe illness.[7] In her original study on the reactions people go through when faced with change, she shows series of states: from an initial shock, through denial, then frustration, anger, and depression, before they begin to reemerge through experimentation, and then reexpression. Though Elisabeth Kubler-Ross first developed this in the late 1960s in relation to breast cancer care, and though it has been taken up by many paramedical and even medical practices since, these ideas were still received as new by politicians, and eagerly explored.

Stephen explained that the process of coming to terms with disability was prolonged and complex, and that people might be as vulnerable some months after their acute event as immediately afterwards. Furthermore, their mood and view of the world might be relatively outgoing while on a hospital ward but they could become quite depressed and isolated once discharged.

He spoke with an authority flowing from his disability. To see him speaking with such power and energy from his chair must have made even the most hardened and selfish politician listen.

In parallel with his talks to employers, he was also running seminars with disabled people. In these they would talk about the experience of disability: its depression, worthlessness, and loss of self-esteem, and ways to overcome this. Stephen described these simply and without emotion, but each time he took a group, he had to revisit his own private experiences, remembering the long periods in Stoke and the countless operations. He was testing his own considerable rehabilitation and recovery as he helped others. He talked of depression as like being in a ditch, unable to see a way out, only able to see the ditch stretching out in both directions. One delegate said that if you stay in a ditch long enough you could be quite comfortable. Another said that a ditch is a grave with the ends kicked out.

Stephen would move on and talk less about the ditch or the depression, and more about the problems of staying in the ditch, either due to depression or dependency, and the need to escape. He made up his approach in the early days of DML as he researched but, most importantly, from his own experience and observation. He had devised his own technique akin to cognitive behavior therapy, or CBT. It was a long way from the medical view of disability and rehabilitation he had been brought up with before his injury. He now realized that there was no easy way, and that each person had to do much himself or herself and take responsibility for their own recovery. They had to recover a control over their lives that had oftentimes, they thought, been taken from them by their injury, and by the expectations of subsequent passivity they learned from medical and other staff.

Stephen explained that many disabled people had adopted or internalized the medical or tragedy model of disability as their truth. Having evolved his own form of CBT to combat his own problems, he developed it more formally for those with spinal cord injury and other disabilities, to encourage them to recover control over their lives.

"What we tried, and try, to do is to conceptualize their disability as being like a stone or stones (since many people have more than one problem). It might be a problem caused by disability, but equally by work, or a relationship with partner, whatever. We get them to quantify their stone and then ask if they can put it down. If they go to the cinema, then can they leave their stone outside? Tinnitus, back pain, they probably can."

Stephen finished his Ph.D. and also built up DML. He was one of a group who, in the United Kingdom, pushed disability issues up the political consciousness. What had begun with his personal observations had led to him being quoted in Parliament and listened to by ministers.

The Gateway Project

A few years ago, Stephen was given some money to work with disabled people in Hampshire and put his theories into practice. Employers would say they would employ more disabled people but that they never turned up for interviews. Disabled people would say they applied for jobs but were turned down before the interview.

Through the Benefits Agency, they unearthed 50,000 people in Hampshire on incapacity benefit. They were unable to contact them directly because of privacy laws, so they advertised in local papers for people who were disabled and who wanted a job. Six hundred people replied, and from these just over four hundred turned up. Stephen and his fellow trainers must have made an odd bunch. One trainer had a false leg, arms that ended at the elbow, and only one hand, due to a congenital problem. He still rode a motorbike and was last heard of running a bar in Thailand.

By employing disabled people where possible, they demonstrated a commitment to practicing what they preached. They also showed their clients, who often had low self-esteem, what disabled people could do, and showed that the project would have good insight into the problem. For Stephen, at last, he was being paid to provide rehabilitation for disabled people. The rub was that he was faced with people who had been indoctrinated to consider themselves the long-term disabled, passive, tragic, demoralized and unemployable, many of whom had been unsuccessfully trying to find work for years on their own.

The series of lectures and courses, which lasted a full nine months, began with a day's seminar explaining the whole project, what they were hoping for and, equally well, what they were expecting from the clients. Then they chipped away, over a four-day course, at the attitudes and motivation of their clients and detailed some of the problems that might prevent someone from working and seeking work. Next they taught people how to manage their searches for jobs, and gave them the practical tools to seek a job. There were small touches, too: pleasant surroundings, good parking, excellent catering, all designed to give clients a sense of worth and value, often for the first time since their injury or disability. Much of the course was less formal and involved support by the trainers for individuals according to their different circumstances. All the time the trainers, in addition to helping them through the process, were trying to empower their clients to take more command of their lives.

They used a star chart, a favorite of Stephen's, to assess each person's life and experience. It deliberately did not focus on the disability but on the person's perception of their life and their success in several areas. Clients were asked to rank or measure how satisfied they were with a variety of aspects of their life and work: motivation and self, interpersonal skills, reliability, resilience and responsibility, work experience, qualifications and skills, personal circumstances, job goal and career management, and finally practical job searching. These allowed them to focus on weaknesses and offer help, as well as reinforcing the positive aspects. Importantly it also allowed them to measure any change in an individual's progress. The charts allowed them a measure of the clients' competence and so allowed them to focus on individuals' problems. Just as important, it allowed the clients some insight into their own abilities and needs.

The official independent report of the trial, which runs to just under two hundred pages, shows that the project exceeded its expectations.[8] Of those who had completed it, roughly 50 percent were likely to have a job. This might not appear a huge effect, but each individual going from "being disabled" to working represents a huge change. The dry report, however, focusses on the economic arguments. The entire project cost £150,000 and is likely to save the government £400,000 over five years as those people lose Incapacity Benefit and become contributors to income tax and national insurance. Scaled up to the country as a whole, such an approach might save £700M per year, or 10 percent of the entire incapacity benefit budget. These are not small figures.

The independent report identified key areas in the success of the project. These were the insight that the barrier to employment was not the disability itself but the attitudes and assumptions that frequently surround it, and that the entire project was conducted on a human scale and by a team with a high proportion of disabled tutors. On the down side, the report focusses on familiar shortcomings, partly in DML and their approaches to the funding bodies and, particularly, that the government departments involved in funding were slow in dealing with matters and so overworked that people were unable to give it sufficient time and thought.

So DML and their partners in the Employment Forum on Disability have shown that something can be done to bring people who are disabled into employment in a financially efficient way, and in a manner that changes people's lives. All the government has to do is spend some money in one department, Education and Employment, to save money in others, Social Services and Health. In the United Kingdom "joined up government" was a mantra; it has—alas—been heard less of late.

Doing Less

By the late 1990s, Stephen had built DML to a £1M turnover per year, offering a wide range of disability services, from the initial advising on disability awareness, to training in disability in employment, and on access issues to work and banks, cinemas, even trains.[9] Stephen had been one of many instrumental in hauling disability up the table of political and social issues in Britain, and while doing all this he developed a company that provided expertise and help in the practical issues that were consequent on these changes.

But as DML enlarged, his ability to control it diminished. He wanted the company to grow. He found a group of non-executive directors with capital, and planned to bring in a managing director and build up DML to another level of profitability. Then it might be sold to a larger company, ideally not in disability, but in insurance or health care, making it more mainstream. But he could not persuade the other members of the senior management team, perhaps because disability affairs and high finance make curious bedfellows. He was also faced with a familiar problem in businesses built on the abilities and drive of a single person: how to grow his company and yet make it appear independent of him. He tried bringing in fresh talent, but still could not convince his fellow directors. At one stage, Stephen thought of closing the business. Then two of his partners offered to buy it.[10] Stephen agreed to give up some parts of the business and concentrate on his interests, disability and management of time away from work, personal development, and expert witness work. He is now free from the business of managing fifteen others and can do what he enjoys, with the happy coincidence that these are the parts that pay better.

"I am out there doing what I enjoy and what I am good at. I hated managing others. Putting it behind me is wonderful. I charge a good but fair rate for my time, and do less."

Proud

Throughout our conversation I had been talking of people who are disabled or people with spinal injury, while Stephen talked of the disabled. I asked what I was supposed to say to avoid offence.

"The disabled bit is important to me. Most disabled people, seriously disabled people that I know, would—and do—refer to themselves as disabled people because they are proud of it. Less significantly disabled people may refer to themselves as people first, but for me, 'Strength in Sisterhood, Glad to be Gay, Black is Beautiful, Proud to be Disabled.' But it is fair to say I have moved beyond that now and am proud to be a parent, a successful business person, though I do not know if that sounds or is conceited, or just satisfied."

It is clear that whatever the disability or challenge that threatens one's selfhood, coming to terms with it requires a huge resource and a huge stubborn pride, a pride in what has been done, with a recognition of the energy and effort required to do it, rather than an overinflated sense of self worth.

But all this sounded stuffy and I could see that Stephen was ill at ease being too introspective. So I enquired about fun, thinking that might be more difficult to recapture.

He seemed to have played some pranks while an in-patient, initially in Stoke as part of a group of young men. However, from our conversation, it seemed to have been less to the forefront more recently. Stephen replied obliquely. He explained that he was planning his biography, with the deliberately ambiguous title, "The Best Half of My Life," inviting the reader to decide which half the title referred to (he had been tetraplegic for exactly twenty-one of his forty-two years). His whole idea was to invite and challenge people to decide which half it was. He expected readers to be split over which half was best, and would be happy whatever they decided.

"I want people to make an exploration of my life and then make their own exploration about their own lives. I used to do amazing things before my injury, though some were so pathetic. The rugby club at medical school had a Road Eaters Club. You bought a curry from a take away, after lots of beer, tipped it out of the container onto the road and then you had to eat it with your tongue.[11]

"Fun, afterwards, took a long time to come through. People have asked lots of times how long did it take to come to terms with the injury. There were a number of critical stages. The first was McColl saying straight away that don't worry, you will be a doctor. Then going back to med school was important, though the osteomyelitis was a set back, but still I was OK. The next stage was when I met all the disabled people in Southampton. Before,

I was Stephen Duckworth, the doctor in the wheelchair, rather than Stephen Duckworth, proud to be disabled. So I got some pride, the pride of being disabled. I was proud to be a doctor, though this was conceited. Now I am just proud to be me, but I had to be proud to be disabled first. A lot of people have never got there.

"Returning to fun, I have always been highly stressed, and at school, coming up to my public school entrance examinations, I thought if I did not get a scholarship that I would not get in. I did not know I could have gone without an award. I was so worried I had psychogenic vomiting and diarrhea. Then I was stressed by medical exams. More recently I have begun to use meditation and reflection at the end of most days to think what I have done well during the day. Some time ago I decided I needed more fun."

Fun seemed to come after the recovery of some sort of balance in his life, after he relaxed a little professionally. To lobby for disability issues, write a doctorate, set up and run a company in a new field, and have a family suggests a driven man. It seemed more difficult to recapture the playfulness and mischievousness of his youth and medical student days. Maybe fun was, for some time, a luxury. Talking with him now, it infused much of what we talked about.

"I remember taking one of my sons, James, aged four, when he had just started mini rugby, to Hamleys [the huge toy shop in Regent's Street in Central London]. On the top floor they had a giant twelve-foot teddy bear dressed as a Beefeater. I whispered in James' ear, 'Go tackle that teddy bear,' and he sped across the floor and tackled it hard and it fell over with toys flying everywhere. Rose turned and said, 'What do you mean by that?' and he said, 'Daddy told me to do it.'"

One chapter of his biography will be entitled "Getting Stuck," recalling the funniest and best places he has been stuck. Many have been in bathrooms when the door was too heavy or the handle jammed.

"I was in a lift in the Treasury once and this blind man came in when I was in an electric chair with handles. He bumped into me, felt round the handles and said, 'Bloody tea trolleys, they are always leaving them in here.' And I said, 'I am not a tea trolley.' And he replied, 'Shit, that's the first time I've heard a tea trolley speak.'"

Maybe it is as well that he is not pushing DML on and on each day as before. Those years were hard, and Stephen does admit to becoming more tired of late. He also thinks spinal cord injury may accelerate some aspects of aging. Recently he did his own personal star chart, writing out his work, Rose, children, community, personal/spiritual development, friends, diet/exercise, family, and parents. In his seminars he asks people how satisfied they are with their commitment to each of these. He has started to use this balance wheel regularly and to use it as a tool to invest time where he feels he needs to most. Time and choice, he told me, are all that any of us truly have. His have, lately, shifted more toward family and personal things.

"I cannot avoid being disabled, and this colors many areas of life, especially in others' perceptions. Beatrice Wright wrote of the spread phenomenon, in which disability spreads through life. If you are wobbly on your feet, then you are considered wobbly intellectually. You are judged on the most visible thing. The apparent appearance of disability spreads into all areas of life. In Bermuda recently I was asked to go around the opposite side of building by a man who said that if his daughter saw me she would have a disabled child. I was contagious. I am constantly being confronted by drunks saying it must be dreadful. The disability is what they see and is the lead. You should do some sociology."

He was probably right. I looked up at Stephen's bookcase and saw several books on wind surfing. He returned to his studies and how he had changed in his approach to patients after his injury.

"If I had been the medical student as before, rather than the guy in the wheelchair, able to empathize with them about being excluded and vulnerable, they would not have felt able to share some of their thoughts and feelings with me, which, in turn, added a huge amount of value to my life. They also felt able to discuss their sex life with me because I was not perceived as a threat."

I was interviewing a man blind from birth once and asked him where he felt he resided, as I reside in my body and particularly in my face, as I see others as their faces to an extent. The man, Peter White, said that he resided in his voice, as did others for him. I asked Stephen where he felt he resided.

"For me it has changed quite recently. For much of the time it has been my head, but lately, through some personal development work I have done, it is much more my heart. I would love to give that impression.

Working with all these disabled unemployed people and seeing the desperate straits they are in has led me this way."

His greatest gift may lie in being an advocate for disabled people to others, and in arguing their cases before employers and politicians. This strength certainly comes from his own experience; sometimes, he told me, people are more impressed if he says nothing. In showing spinal cord injury without threat to others and in an open approachable way—by humanizing it—Stephen has allowed people to deal with their own concerns. He has reduced the distance between those in chairs and those not, so allowing other people a degree of shared understanding that may be a necessary first step to assisting.

Many of us become set in our goals and careers fairly early on and show a single mindedness in their pursuit. Despite his spinal cord injury and being really only able to move one arm and hand—poorly—Stephen has moved enormous distances in how he views himself and his roles and work. Initially, by his own words, he was a fairly typical and unthinking medical student. Becoming a patient made him confront aspects of himself and, indeed, of life he would probably never have understood or realized. Soon after becoming tetraplegic, once he had the hurdles of qualification in medicine over, he left a clinical life to study disability and its relation to "normal" experience. This may have been in part motivated by knowing just how hard clinical work would be from a chair. But there was something else, something more important.

Within medicine he had to accept the medical model of his injury: it was labelled tragic, catastrophic, and permanent. It was perhaps the ultimate loss—of movement, and of independence. He was expected to be looked after and be grateful for the care offered lovingly and with the best intentions; to be an object and to be passive. In leaving medicine, he cast that aside and explored other ways of looking at his condition and himself. To avoid the tragic view it was imperative that he did leave medicine, for medicine was then capable of viewing him and his condition in only one—pitiable—way.

He became a disability terrorist, within the radical and protesting tradition within the United Kingdom. He became part of a new peer group, and explored new ideas and new ways of living. He became proud to be disabled. Then, after his visit to Australia, his approach to disability changed quite markedly once more. He had to break from others again, this time from the new orthodoxy of disability studies, to work hard on his new ideas of working with politicians and providers, seeking to influence them not from the street with banners but from their own rooms with cogent arguments and with the authority that came from his chair. Unashamedly he used his new position to become part businessman, part politician, and part advocate. He helped bring about changes in disability awareness and provision while building DML to become an established leader in the field. Now, though his vision of the company was thwarted, he is still more active than most people, concentrating more on his smaller chosen fields of disability awareness and legal work. Stephen has certainly been one of those whose work and example have changed the outlook of many other people, including the disabled and the powerful. Once proud to qualify as a doctor, and then proud to be disabled, he is now happy to be Stephen, father, husband, businessman, and guy who goes down to the pub on the weekend.

Soon after he was injured, he had sought the advice of someone in the disability arena. This man had suggested he stay in medicine and seek to change through his example. There seems little doubt that Stephen's influence would not have been as wide or deep if he had.

"My disability can be used as a weapon or a tool. If you've got it, flaunt it. It has taken me to lots of areas and opened many doors. I would not have chosen it, but I have used it once it is there. It has completely altered my outlook on life and, I think, made me a better person."

Who knows what Stephen would have done if he had not made that rugby tackle. Perhaps he'd be a prosperous surgeon with a big yacht, or a primary care physician and captain of the golf club. Either way, it is difficult imaging that he would have questioned his profession and society as much as he has.

In the next chapter is the narrative of someone from a far less privileged background, who dropped out of school to a dead end job and who lived for boozy weekends. His future was poor, even before he broke his neck.

14 Flyers and Nonflyers

A Working-Class Yobbo

The only son of working-class parents, Mike Oliver passed the examinations at eleven for the local grammar school. But the education on offer did not engage him, and he left five years later with only three of the ten O levels expected, branded a failure. A dead-end clerical job followed, as his life centered around cricket, football, and macho weekends with friends. At seventeen, with five of his friends, he went to a holiday camp in Essex. There he dived into a swimming pool and broke his neck.

"I did not know what I had done. My only recollection was that I was obsessed with my legs sticking up in front of me, and I kept saying, 'Put my legs down, put them down.' I was reassured by a Redcoat [a camp attendant] by the pool that it was temporary cramp and that it would go very soon."

It did not. He was taken to the local hospital and his neck stabilized by traction through the skull, possibly one of the most painful experiences of his life—he was only given local anesthetic because of his condition. When he was transferred to Stoke Mandeville two days later, the first thing the boss, Sir Ludwig Guttmann, said was that this man does not need traction.

"Guttmann. It is a major irony in the relationship between major world events and individual biography that while I am probably alive today because of what he brought to the treatment of people with spinal cord injury, he—himself a refugee from one of the greatest dictators the world has ever seen [Hitler]—ran Stoke like a great dictator, and for some it was not a pleasant experience."

Mike, as we will see, has merged his individual experience with political ideas and ideals. He has also written of his experiences and the way they have guided his thoughts, in several books and many articles. I tried to defend Guttmann by suggesting that things were different after the war and that, after all, he did say that his aim was for paraplegics to get back to work. He saw self-esteem tied to employment through work. Mike agreed to a point.

"Yes. All the time I knew him he was obsessed with tetraplegics being able to type. That was the passport to the universe. When I met him for the last time before he died I was a lecturer with my own secretary, and he said, 'How you doing, my boy?' And I said, 'Very well, thank you.' He asked what I did, and I told him. He said, 'Very good, what is your typing speed?' I don't think he moved on. The greatest thing I learned from him was to avoid medical intervention as much as possible. Allow the body to heal itself. It was almost radical nonintervention. I think the body is best left alone and only intervene when you really have to, and that has kept me in good stead."[1]

Mike continued, "I was complete C6/C7. I don't think I was ever given that diagnosis. My recollection is that I was never told I would never walk again, I was never told that was it. Everything I knew I picked up.

"I was a working-class yobbo, doing a dead-end job in an office I did not like. I did not like where my life was going. Once I got out of bed, after three months, the experience was much more like the experience I would have had if conscription to the army had been still in. You worked hard during the day at physio and occupational therapy, and you played at night. You went to the pub each night and had a few drinks. There were lots of accessible women there. Prior to my accident I had never been successful with women . . . like most young men I found women unexplainable and my experience with girls had been not very happy or successful. Here there were women, many of whom were part of the unofficial curriculum, to rehabilitate you in whatever ways it was necessary to rehabilitate you in the evenings once the uniforms had come off.

"I think it is not common knowledge but, nevertheless, particularly the therapists and OTs were encouraged to liase with the patients in a personal as well as professional way. Ironically, I fell foul of that, being only seventeen or eighteen. I actually developed a relationship with a young Irish student nurse, about my age, and that was frowned upon. If I had been going out with a twenty-four-year-old therapist (who could have controlled the relationship), that would have been OK. As it was we spent most of the romance dodging matrons and sisters."

I wondered if the experience of living with spinal cord injury made him more concerned about the other and so attractive for that reason.

"Gosh, it would be nice to think that was true, and I would like to think that, as someone who experiences life as a disabled person. I am not sure it was true at the beginning either for me or the guys round us. Women were there to be used as men have always used women. . . . The idea that disabled men, or even men, as we mature, become more sensitive to the needs of another I think happens to some people whether disabled or not. But for most of us, whether disabled or not, a sense of respecting the needs of others passes us by."

Stage Theory?

Mike has argued in several articles against a coming to terms with the loss he experienced. He denies stages of anger or guilt or depression.

"It had happened and I had to get on with it. That is not to say, on occasions, that I did not become angry or depressed. But what I have written against is that these feelings are generated by the paralysis itself, that you have this traumatic event which results in loss and this generates the need to go through a series of stages. That is too mechanical, and it takes people out of their social context.

"I was angry when I was discharged, but I was angry not because I had not come to terms with my spinal injury, as I am sure the social worker that used to visit me would have written in her case notes. I was angry because I had to eat, sleep, and defecate in the same room, and that was the room I shared with my parents when we watched television as well.

"My work has been not an attempt to dismiss the feeling we all have as human beings in the situations we find ourselves, but to criticize the view that people have to be pigeon-holed like that, and that if they do not go through that process then they can never be properly psychologically healed or whole. I think that is nonsense."

Mike had written on this adjustment previously: "When something happens to an individual's body something happens to the mind as well. To become fully human again, in order to form a disabled identity, the disabled individual must undergo medical treatment and physical rehab, as well as the process of psychological adjustment or coming to terms with. They must grieve and mourn his lost ability and pass through a series of stages. However, the conceptual framework has been severely criticized, on theoretical and existential grounds."[2]

He finds little evidence for such simple, consecutive stages, quoting Zola:

I realise how meagre are our attempts to write and do research about adjustment and adaptation. It would be nice if, at some point, growing up ends and maturity begins, or if one could say that successful adjustments and adaptations to a particular difficulty has been achieved. For most problems, or perhaps most basic life issues, there is no single time for such a resolution. . . . The problems must be faced, evaluated, re-defined, and readapted to, again and again and again. And I knew that this applied to myself. No matter how much I was admired by others or by myself, there was still much more I had to face. "My Polio" and "My Accident" were not just my past: they were part of my present and my future.[3]

In expecting patients to conform to models of psychological adjustment, health care professionals reinforce the lie, Mike suggested.

"Some say you are in denial, and the more you deny, the more the denial. A silly argument you just cannot win. I think I was a sociologist before I knew I was. Most of the people I kind of spent time with, watching them go through all the experience, did not go through all of that either. Certainly not in the way that academics suggest."

Elisabeth Kubler-Ross wrote her seminal and very influential work[4] after a relatively short time in a clinical unit, only two and a half years of working with patients with breast cancer. I wondered why he thought her theories had such agreement and acceptance.

"Because they lock into the dominant model and perception of spinal cord injury [and other impairments]: that spinal cord injury is a personal tragedy. It's as simple as that. As an able-bodied person you look at what has happened and you say, 'Broken your neck, lost sensation, no movement, no control of bladder and bowels, as well as not being able to walk,' and think how awful that is.

"That there are periods of mourning and denial, of anger and then restoration allows others to move on from the impairment and, after a while, put it behind them and expect the patient to as well."

For Mike this is such an oversimplification and distortion. It does not conform to what he has felt, nor what he has found in most others in the same situation. People may come to terms with, but never forget or put behind them severe life events. But that is not to say that people's responses don't change with changing circumstances.

"A month before I had had my accident, I had gone to a dance and I spent the whole of the evening talking with a guy I met who was in a wheelchair. (I had gone with a girl, but halfway through I was not with her any more for some reason.) I was feeling a bit sorry for myself, since everyone else was up dancing, so I went to talk to him. I remember clearly thinking after that that if it ever happened to me I could not stand it. I would want to kill myself, and I was upset about it for days.

"But once it did happen to me, all the things I thought I would think and feel, I never felt at all. I take from that the lesson that we are not able truly to know ourselves, however well we think we do. If someone dies, or we go home and our partner says they are divorcing us, or we lose our job, though we might have thought about those things before and how we might think, I do not think any of us really knows how we would feel beforehand."

Acquiring a disability is to abandon all our preconceptions.

Pure Chance

I returned to his time in Stoke. He must have had extensive physiotherapy and occupational therapy during his time there?

"Most of what I learned that was useful I learned from people with spinal cord injury. Most of what I learned from therapists, OTs, and nurses was how to get on with members of the opposite sex. Even things like how to get in and out of cars I learned from other disabled people. How to put my own trousers on, how to put on my condom incontinence device, I learned from watching other people.

"I was discharged. I could have come out a couple of months earlier, but we were waiting for a bed and some adaptations, but these did not occur. Stoke got so fed up that they discharged me and said go home and manage, or go to the local general hospital. The irony is that the situation has not changed in forty years. It seems there is no way to speed this up unless you have money.

"I did not want to go home. I was having a great time; hard work during the day, in physio. I would get stood up every day so I would be in a close proximity to young women. If I was at home, where was I going to get all this from? Then OT and archery and table tennis, then out to the pub in the evenings. And I had that relationship with a young nurse. I was quite happy. I would still be there now, still drinking. . . .

"I think I learned more about myself and personal relationships in the one year I spent there than I have in the twenty years in another kind of institution, the university. Other important gains . . . relationships with parents and other family members grew stronger at a time when often for young people such relationships grow weaker. On leaving, mates and working-class community welcomed me back.[5]

"But I was discharged and spent a few months living in one room until eventually the accommodation was built at home. I spent the next two years at home being unemployed, being visited by the social worker every three months. I was very fed up and thought I was unemployable. I had no idea what I could do. I had completely internalized what I had been taught. I could type thirty words per minute, like Guttmann had asked."

Mike has written of this time, "For a while all was well. My life continued as it had before except that I did not have a boring clerical job. . . . Soon it became apparent that endless days without boring work were even more boring than endless days with it. . . . I began to feel . . . that there must be more to life than watching television and being taken out by your mates and drinking."[6]

This might have gone on for years more, with Mike expecting to do nothing, being expected to do nothing. But then a stroke of pure chance altered his expectations.

"I lived in a little village called Borstal, which housed the first ever Borstal Institution [for young offenders].[7] While I had been in Stoke, I had met a guy from the same village who was a paraplegic in his fifties who had been a prison officer at the Borstal. Previously he was a farm worker and had been driving his tractor when it turned over and broke his back. The Prison Service then created a job for him as a clerk in the library. When he came up for retirement, the principal of the Education Centre said to him that they had got used to having him around and that the place was laid out for a wheelchair user. 'We still need someone to do your job. Do you know anyone in the village?'

"Bill mentioned me, and the next thing I know is that I am lying in bed at 10:30 one morning, since there is nothing to get up for, and I am waiting for my Mum to come with my cup of tea and bacon sandwich, when there is a knock on the door. A very strangely dressed guy with long hair, before it was fashionable, asked, 'Is Michael in?' My Mum said, 'Yes.' 'Well I've come to see him.' 'But you can't, he's in bed.' And he said, 'That doesn't matter,' and sort of pushed his way into the house and said to me, 'What are you doing?' and I said, 'Lying in bed.' He said, 'Do you want a job?' and I said, 'Yes, I think so.' So he said, 'OK, I'll come to pick you up on Monday, we need a clerk up at the Institution, and I'll come and pick you up.' I said, 'But what I am going to do, and how I am going to get there, and I have not got a car.' He said, 'Don't worry about this, I'll sort it out.'

"For the next four months, either he or another officer or a teacher would pick me up in the morning and I would do whatever work was needed. It took me a while to learn to write again. Then one of the staff would take me home. That went on for a few months. Then this guy, Peter, said, 'I am not coming to pick you up forever you know.' So I said, 'I know that.' 'It is time you got a car.' I said, 'I can't afford one. I have not got the money, the job is only a part-time one.' He said, 'Well the job is there as long as you want it.' So I managed to borrow some money and opened a bank account, and passed my driving test and got a car."

From Literacy to Sociology

"A few months later—well six months or a year—he came to see me again. 'We've got too many lads in and not enough people to teach them. How do you feel about taking a couple of classes?' I said, 'In what?' 'Nothing special, just sit in with them and listen to them read and help them.' So I started taking classes in basic numeracy and literacy, and then I would go in and find I was timetabled for this and that, general studies, sex education, and, before I knew it, I had a full-time job as a lecturer in the establishment. I had gone from being a rotten clerk to being a lecturer without noticing it.

"I did that for three years, and then I had another Peter moment. He called me into his office, since by then we had moved and he had a posh office. He said, 'You can't stay here forever you know.' I said, 'Why not?' He said, 'A, it's not healthy, and B, the government have just changed the regulations and in a couple of years time I will not be able to employ people without a formal qualification. So you had better make up your mind what you are doing with the rest of your life.' So I kind of thought about it, and he said, 'I think you should go to teacher trainer's college.'

"But by then I did not feel I had been stretched. My survival technique during these first three years, when I was teaching various subjects—by the end I was teaching A level history and citizenship—was that I would go to night school and be one week ahead of what I was teaching. I discovered at night school that the University of Kent, which had just opened in the late '60s, had this course in sociology, and I looked at the syllabus and thought it would help me with my teaching history and citizenship. So I enrolled.

"That grabbed me. For the first time in my life I actually found something academic which spoke to me, and from then on I had this relationship with sociology. It grabbed me by the balls and it has never let go. So when he said, 'You need a qualification, go away and train as a teacher,' I thought, 'Stuff that, I will become a sociologist.'

"I went to university, which was also my escape from my parents. They were getting older, and my Dad had just retired, and I realized that both for good and bad reasons that I did not want to live the rest of life with them. I needed my space and they needed theirs. They had worked hard all their lives, and if I went out on a Saturday night, then they had to wait up until 3 a.m. for me to come and to put me back to bed. It was partly an opportunity to sort out my own life. That was the next break. I met my first wife, went to university, and got my Ph.D.

"Peter lives in Wales, and we still exchange Christmas cards and ring each other up every so often. Without him I could not have broken the vicious circle of needing a car to get a job and needing money to buy a car. In a sense that has changed with mobility allowance. But there were lots of young men who never worked because of this. I don't see that as me being superior, I was just lucky. He believed in everyone, even the vilest of the young kids in the Borstal, even those who went on to perform the vilest of murders. But Peter believed. Whether he was a Christian Socialist or whatever, he saw the best in people."

It seemed that he gave, or allowed, Mike time to explore and discover the beginnings of self-respect at a time when it had been wrenched from him by his accident and by what had happened subsequently.

"You and I would intellectualize this now, but that is not what happened. At the time, he gave me a job and he gave me money. That meant I could buy a Ford Cortina, and that meant I could go out by myself on a Saturday evening. That meant, in turn, that I could go back to what I had been quite good at, picking up women. Out of that, a good sense of self-esteem might have emerged. But he was not consciously building my self-confidence; he gave me a car and access to women."

Mike was awakened, passionately, by exposure to education and to sociology. But this is not to suggest that his education was easy. For the most part it was just the opposite, mainly because of the physical difficulties of access he had to overcome in the early 1970s. He had talked almost as though once he started education his physical impairment was irrelevant. But being in a wheelchair was never irrelevant.

"When I went to night school for O level math or history, I was told I could not go in. They did not allow people like me in; I was told I might be a fire hazard. There were no toilets. I had to drive outside and then bully and cajole people to help me in. I would use my car horn to get someone to help me."

"Higher education was not welcoming. For those few disabled people in it in the early 1970s, it was a real struggle. Psychoanalysts might say that maybe it was my hidden anger driving me on, and I don't know. Part of it might have come from Peter, and part from Bob Dylan, who opened me up to notions of justice. I knew I had a right to be in night school and university. I would be there whether they wanted me or not, so there was a sense of bloody mindedness.

"Going to a seminar in a four-story-high building where there were no lifts on a Tuesday afternoon, I would sit at the bottom of the stairs and wait till there were four students who would carry me up for sociological theory. Now automatically people with disability problems are timetabled with some help, but at no time then was being in a wheelchair irrelevant."

I waffled about how some people with spinal cord injury are always aware of their impairment. I should have known by now that Mike would disagree.

"I never saw it in those terms. It was that I was pissed off that I had to be lifted up stairs, and then going between buildings there might be an incline and I would wait for a pretty girl and ask for a push, and then you could ask if they wanted a drink or whatever. So it was a passport to riches as well as being a pain in the ass. It is neither one thing nor the other; it can be both almost at the same time."

Consensus and Conflict

I asked of his intellectual development and how he had moved into the sociology of disability.

"Sociology was perceived as being radical then, though it was not. There were two ways of viewing the world: in consensual terms and conflict terms . . . but a lot of the structures of academia were still in place. I was discouraged from disability work since I would not be able to be objective, that great academic god of impartiality. My main interest, as an undergraduate, was crime and deviancy. My Ph.D. was on the sociological aspects of epilepsy. What interested me was that during my time at Borstal, nearly every week there would be someone who had a major fit, a "wobble" they used to call it in the Nick. Yet I had never met or seen anyone have a fit outside. What was it about prisons which made people have wobbles inside?

"I looked at three groups of young men with epilepsy, one in Borstal, one in a psychiatric hospital—and I did some work at the Maudsley— and one in the community. It was from a prospective of crime and deviance, not health and illness. But since epilepsy is medical, I had to get into the medical stuff, and when I started to read it I could not believe how unrelated it was to my experience and the experience of those I knew. There seemed to be a whole industry in which people were writing about us and our lives in ways which made absolutely no sense whatever, and were not about our problems and experiences at all. This was at the time when feminism was beginning to appear on campuses, and I would go along to learn their perspective and get thrown out, women only. I would say, I am on your side, I want to learn more, and

I want to know how the personal is the political, and they would say, 'Piss off, you're a man.' "

I related how I was involved with a play, Peter Brook's *L'Homme Qui*, based on Oliver Sacks' book of the same name. At one workshop, Peter had been asked by a woman why the actors were all men. He looked pained. "There are women on stage, but they are played by men." The feminist was silent.

"The combination of the influence of feminist writings and my own disbelief about what was being written in the medical literature set me off with a burning desire to change all that."

He was fortunate again in that around that time the new distance-learning organization, the Open University, was looking for tutors for a new course in disability. In applying, it was an advantage to be disabled. With a wife and young family to support, he needed employment, and this was the ideal job. Not only was he able to teach, but also around him were other influential figures in the new-ish disability movement aiming to change perceptions and improve the lives of those with various disabilities.

Vic Finkelstein, for instance, also living with spinal cord injury, had railed against the injustice, falsity, and wrong headedness of some of the rehabilitation he was made to follow:

The aim of returning the individual to normality is the central foundation stone on which the whole rehabilitation machine is constructed. If, as happened to me following my spinal injury, the disability cannot be cured, normative assumptions are not abandoned. On the contrary, they are re-formulated so that they not only dominate the treatment phase searching for a cure, but also totally colour the helper's perception of the rest of that person's life. The rehabilitation aim now becomes to assist the individual to be "as normal as possible."

The result, for me, were endless soul-destroying hours at Stoke Mandeville Hospital trying to approximate to able-bodied standards by "walking" with callipers and crutches. . . . Rehabilitation philosophy emphasises physical normality and, with that, the attainment of skills that allow the individual to approximate as closely as possible to able-bodied behaviour (e.g., only using a wheelchair as a last resort, rather than seeing it as a disabled peoples' mobility aid like a pair of shoes is an able-bodied person's mobility aid).[8]

The OU course was not on handicapped persons but on "The Disabling Society." Disability was due not to illness, but because of the social barriers, restrictions, and/or oppressions people with impairments face, and the professional interventions have come to be seen as often adding to these problems, rather seeking to deal with them.

Over the succeeding years, Mike taught, wrote, and lectured, refining and defining his ideas. Dissatisfied with a purely academic or intellectual role, he served on various committees for both health care provision with other professionals, but also for the Spinal Injuries Association—run by and for those with spinal injury. For the first few years after his injury, even while at the Borstal, he had seen others with spinal injury during sports events or socially and had met few people with other impairments. As he did meet people with a variety of problems, he gained a political awareness as well as a career. These led to a growing involvement with disabled people and in organizations created to advance their views and opportunities.

In the mid 1990s, he became the first, and so far only, professor of disabilities studies in Britain, at the University of Greenwich.[9] Typically, in his inaugural address, he discussed something he had not done for over thirty years, walking. He divided the world not into able and disabled people, but into walkers, nonwalkers, and nearly walkers—those encouraged and cajoled, he said, by health care professionals to attempt something inherently difficult, hazardous, and of marginal utility.

He discussed the popular songs equating walking tall with manliness and vigor, he satirized organizations claiming that cure for spinal cord injury was close to hand, and he made the case for the validity of living from a chair.

"We do not punish nonflyers for not flying, why punish nonwalkers? We spend billions of dollars making mobility aids for nonflyers, called planes, airports, and runways. Millions of people are employed to help nonflyers to overcome their mobility difficulties, environments are degraded and destroyed.

"True, all people are nonflyers, but the numbers who fly worldwide are actually smaller than the nonwalkers or nearly walkers."[10]

It must have been a far cry from the usual inaugural lectures giving a potted history of the new professor's brilliant research career to date.

The Best Thing That Had Ever Happened to Me

Mike has not confined his writing to journals and books, though these have been his main output. His academic articles have been criticized for being difficult for general readers. In discussing the sociological issues around disability he has also avoided personal problems. As ever, he meets criticism head on: "My own response is that . . . understanding disability requires a great deal of intellectual effort. If we are going to transform ourselves and society it is only we, as disabled people, who can do the necessary intellectual work.

"As far as the absence of a personal or subjective dimension, there are two reasons. There is a thin line between writing subjectively and exposing things which are and should remain private. . . . There is [also] danger in emphasizing the personal at the expense of the political, because most of the world still thinks of disability as an individual, intensely personal problem."[11]

He avoids the personal where possible, but not always, and his writing is not all in academic outlets. In 1984, he wrote a famous article for the newspaper *The Guardian*.

I had been talking to him about the different lives people must lead before and after injury. My drift may have been to give a value to each and explore what is possible in this. I may have implicitly intimated a value judgement. Mike took me up on this.

"About not worse, not different—there is a third difference—that SCI makes life better. That is why I wrote the piece in *The Guardian* about my disability being the best thing that had ever happened to me. Because—for me—I think it was. I was a working-class yobbo with a failed education, not very good at relationships, in a job that I did not like, and I probably would have gone on to drink too much. . . . I was a promising sportsman but had failed in that, too. I was a smoker.

"Breaking my neck broke that mold and gave me an alternative possibility. It changed the possibility of whom I could become. Forty years later, I am a professor of disability studies, I have one marriage behind me and I am happily married again. I have grandchildren and have been all over the world. I have had a good life. I have no complaints. One thing I do know, that if I had not broken my neck, I would not be a professor in a university. But equally well, I do not want to be positioned as some sort of hero, who struggled against appalling circumstances. I have just taken opportunities as they occurred.

"After that article about disability being the best thing that happened to me, you would be amazed by the flack that I got from a huge range of people. Some disabled, some not. I was accused of being mad or telling lies to get in the paper. As a result of this, I was invited to go on a pop medical program that went out, live, *Where's There's Life*. At the time it attracted 18 million people, not because it was a wonderful program but because it was just before Coronation Street [the most popular soap]. Miriam Stoppard, the interviewer, clearly could not understand or handle what I tried to say in the piece. She tried to get me to admit that what I said was untrue and false, and that I really did feel that something tragic had happened.

"In the end, after ten minutes of sparring verbally she said, 'Look, there's Mount Everest out there and you will never be able to climb it.' It was one of those times when normally in an argument you remember three hours later what you should have said, but for some reason out of my head, I looked at her and said, 'Miriam, look, the four-minute mile is out there, and you will never be able to run it, so why do you assume that my life is a tragedy and yours isn't?'

"The general point was that all of us have a relationship between our body and our environment, and the relationship between these two allows us to do some things and does not allow us to do other things. I do not want in some way for disabled people to be considered different, because all we are doing is trying to make sense of that experience in the same ways that you do. Where we are different, because I do not want to deny difference either, is that whereas society takes cognizance of your needs in relation with the environment, it does not take cognizance of our needs. Often it goes out of its way to prevent our needs being met. You can jump onto a bus or plane easily. I cannot."

The Importance of Definitions

In his work and those of many others in the "disability movement," Mike has sought to redefine the terms and, more importantly, the perceptions of disability. As he suggests, definitions are not unimportant, for "the social human world differs from the natural one in that humans give meanings to objects in the social world and subsequently orientate their behavior toward those objects in terms of the meanings given to them."[12]

So if disability is seen as a tragedy, then disabled people will be treated as if they are passive victims. This will not only affect the way they see themselves, but also be transferred into social policy. Mike and others suggest another model. Though initially arising from sociology and not medicine, their ideas have become more and more accepted and form the underpinning of an important document from the Royal College of Physicians of London and The Prince of Wales' Advisory Group on Disability.[13] It offers the following definitions:

Impairment is the loss or abnormality of a particular faculty or part of the body.

Someone with a disabling impairment is a disabled person.

Disability refers to a disabled person's encounter with daily living, the environment and society, not only in particular circumstances but encompassing the whole of that experience.

This is all presaged in Mike's 1990 book, *The Politics of Disability:*

The individual model [of disability] sees the problem as stemming from the functional limitations or psychological losses assumed to arise from disability, underpinned by the personal tragedy model of disability, suggesting in turn that disability is some terrible chance event occurring at random to unfortunate individuals. Nothing could be further from the truth.

The social model suggests it is not the disability, not individual limitations, which are the cause of the problem but society's failure to provide appropriate services and failure to ensure the needs of disabled people are fully taken into account.

Hence disability is all the things which impose restrictions on disabled people, from individual prejudice to institutional discrimination, to inaccessible buildings to unusable transport systems.[14]

In this Mike is suggesting that the medical aspects of his impairment are manageable and that it is all the problems heaped on him by society in terms of access and employment that are more important. Not surprising, some have protested that such a model ignores the medical problems that would remain even if all social disability was removed. "Sometimes . . . proponents of independent living have tended to discuss disablement as if it had nothing to do with the physical body."[15]

For Mike, however, this is not a problem and, indeed, is given within the definitions:

Ironically that is precisely what the social model insists, disablement is nothing to do with the body. It is a consequence of social oppression. But the social model does not deny impairment is closely related to the physical body. Impairment is, in fact, nothing less than a description of the physical body.

The social model does not deny that some illnesses have disabling consequences. . . . Doctors have to treat the impairment and its consequences, but they are no good at disability. . . . The whole medical and rehabilitation enterprise is founded upon an ideology of normality . . . to restore the disabled person to normality. Where that is not possible, the basic aim is not abandoned; the goal is to restore the disabled person to a state that is as near normality as possible. So surgical intervention and physical rehabilitation, whatever its costs in terms of pain and suffering of disabled individuals. . . .

Further, the medical profession, because of its power and dominance, has spawned a whole range of pseudo-professions in its own image: physiotherapy, OT, etc., each geared to its own normality.[16]

Acceptance of these ideas requires a huge perceptual shift. For Mike and others the problems with living with spinal cord injury are mainly social ones, to do with lack of access and lack of independence, and have little to do with the physical embodied impairment. This they can live with and care not to focus upon. What they want and need are more opportunities to live as the rest of us do in terms of work, recreation, mobility, pay, and so on.[17]

"There can be only two possible explanations why disabled people experience a quality of life so much poorer that everyone else: one, that disability has such a traumatic physical and psychological effect on individuals that they cannot ensure a reasonable quality of life or themselves by their own efforts; the other, that the economic and social barriers that disabled people face are so pervasive that [they] are prevented from ensuring themselves a reasonable quality of life by their own efforts."[18]

For Mike, the first has been assumed far too long. For Mike, a Marxist, the economic and social barriers reflect the marginalization of nonproductive people with the onset of industrialization.

"For me, the main reason why disabled people are discriminated against is the Big C—capitalism. It's directly linked to the industrial mode of production. That required particular kinds of bodies, and disabled people did not fit that mold, and we then became excluded from that workforce, which presented all kinds of problems. That meant we were considered dis-abled, unable to contribute. We then became social problems and required governments to respond to these problems. You cannot have these on the streets, so policies have to be created to get them off the streets, so they do it in terms of institutions.

"Disabled people were institutionalized as a warning to others. If you do not conform to what Foucault termed 'the disciplinary regime,' then you will end up in an institution, and institutions deliberately set out to provide a quality of life worse than if you had lived outside, however poor you were."

I had come a long way during our afternoon together, and Mike given me much to think about. He gave me another book and a reading list on my way out. As I walked back to the station, I imagined myself in a wheelchair, negotiating all the bumps in the pavements, the curbs without cuts, the steps down to the station, and the turnstile at the platform entrance. I normally passed through this world without attention toward it. Now I could see it, see the problems with access and realize how disabled people could feel excluded. I still needed time, though, to see it as social oppression.

15 | Empowerment

The Political and Personal

Both Mike and Stephen responded to their injuries with huge invention. Mike has gone on record that it was the best thing that has happened to him, while Stephen suggests that his injury has made him a better, more perceptive person. They have both gone beyond their own injuries to contribute hugely to the debates around disability and to social policy to improve provisions, not only for those with spinal cord injury but also for all disabled in Britain. Their differing backgrounds may have had some influence on the differing paths they have chosen.

Stephen, though he flirted with the disability movement, thought he would be more effective and warmer if he were in the room with the politicians and policymakers rather than in the street protesting. This has led to him gaining the ear of politicians, to power meals with ministers, and even to his Ph.D. thesis being quoted in Parliament. He has argued from the individual to the general, using the experiences of a few to argue for alterations in laws and attitudes. He has done this with a conciliatory style and from a broadly capitalist stance, whether talking to governments of the right or left. He has made them realize that people with impairments who are independent and working cost less in the long run than dependent, unemployed disabled people.

He has used his own personal charm and savvy, being least radical and most consensual with junior people, the gatekeepers of the high-up policymakers and company directors. Once he has gained access to the board rooms and cabinets, then his personal charm and authority persist, but with more openness and radical ideas.

When I asked Stephen how best to help disabled people, his first thought, half jokingly, was to take their benefits away. Without the expectation of state support, without the strings of dependence, people with disability would expect to work and carry on their lives as best they could, despite and with their impairment. As importantly, he would hope that, if without benefits, the able bodied would not be encouraged to think of disabled people as dependent. For Stephen the way back is employment. He has spent much of his professional life arguing for, and finding ways of, helping people with disability into employment, whether through disability awareness seminars for businessmen and politicians, workshops helping with interview technique and self-esteem for prospective disabled employees, or through the grind of helping to make buildings and public transport accessible. Along the way he has also made a living and raised a family.

This would have delighted Sir Ludwig Guttmann. When he set up Stoke Mandeville hospital, his main aim was "to transform a hopeless and helpless spinally injured paralyzed individual into a tax payer."

He was concerned to explain that "although this might, on first hearing, sound rather materialistic, in fact it is the ultimate aim of rehabilitation. For such a person can look anybody straight in the eye and say 'I am as good as you, and perhaps even a little better, for to become a taxpayer in my condition, wheelchair-bound for life, I have first had to overcome one of the greatest tragedies in the human condition.'"[1]

Note Guttmann's use of the tragic.

Michael, in contrast to Stephen, has remained more on the outside. He's been not so much on the street with a banner but certainly within a loose disability movement, a union of those with various impairments, convinced of the need to band together to be heard. He has used his academic interest to guide his practical work. In his book *Understanding Disability*, he describes this in terms of a movement from the personal to the political. For Mike, a disabled individual who lives completely apart from others with similar and differing impairments is more likely to see her- or himself in personal and tragic terms. By meeting others with similar and different impairments comes a realization of how unnecessary and destructive a tragic model of impairment is. From a sense of community with others with impairments, individuals may gain self-respect otherwise denied them. If attitudes and laws are to be changed, then it is only through such bandings together that pressure can be exerted on the lawmakers and on society as a whole; and only disabled people can do it. A social model is necessary to avoid the medical tragedy model of disability, to free individuals from its consequences and to allow change.

Dependent

Both Stephen and Michael question the concept of independence. Stephen often asks about it at workshops.

"'I am independent.' What does that mean? I often ask that of delegates in a seminar. I say stick your hand up if you traveled here independently today? And everyone puts his or her hands up. Then I ask how many came by train, and half put their hand up, and I ask, 'OK, how many of you built the train?'"

"They talk this through, and they eventually realize that they may need the contribution of up to a million people to get through the day, with train operators, train makers, track fitters, maintenance men, electricity workers, even before those involved with the manufacture of their clothes and food are considered.

"We are all dependent. Those with spinal cord injury are no different to others. The concept of independence, meaning doing it for your self, is misguided and simplistic and does enormous harm."

Mike agrees. "I do not subscribe to a notion of dependent and independent. We are all mutually dependent, and we are some of us physically dependent on others and others are emotionally dependent on us. When we are talking about those relationships, I do not think it helps to talk about them in single terms. We have family members, friends, lovers, sons, and daughters. Why do we position people in relation to others and what they do?

"When my first wife left, she left not only me but also two teenage children. According to the literature, they were young carers in need of protection. The reality was that they did nothing for me, that was all done by PAs. Sometimes I would come home at night and the music would be going so loud that they would not even hear me on the drive, so they would not bring my wheelchair out. I had to stop people on the street and say, 'Here's my key, could you pop in the house and get my wheelchair?'

"But they were completely dependent on me physically. Without me paying someone to do the shopping, they would have starved, yet I am reading that there are these young people left with a single parent and seen as carers."

Whereas Stephen has worked with and reached many individuals through his work and has sought change through such meetings, for Mike the individual is less to the fore, at least in his theoretical work. He thinks that personal tragedy theory has individualized the problems of disability and so tended to leave social and economic structures untouched. For him another, social, model was necessary.

The Private and the Public

Neither Michael nor Stephen is inclined to dwell on their own impairments; Stephen talks about his medical management but less about his personal details. Michael rarely mentions his impairment. Understandably for people whose work places them in a public position, they guard their privacy. But there is more to it. If they did focus on their neurological impairment, it would focus on them personally when they want to broaden the issue to social models of disability.

Mike's article in *The Guardian* was strongly criticized by a woman with spinal cord injury for whom the day-to-day inconveniences of the condition were a constant trial and for whom Mike's article, all but ignoring them, was almost incomprehensible. Jenny Morris, a disabled woman and author, also picked up on this:

There is a tendency within the social model of disability to deny the experience of our own bodies, insisting that our physical differences and restrictions are entirely socially created. While environmental barriers and social attitudes are a crucial part of our experience of disability—and do indeed disable us—to suggest that this is all there is to it is to deny the personal experience of physical or intellectual restrictions, of illness, of dying.[2]

Liz Crow has also argued that we need to integrate the experience of impairment and that of disability. Up to now the social model has insisted that there is no causal relationship between the two: "The achievement of the disability movement has been to break the link between our bodies and our social situation, and to focus on the real cause of disability, i.e., discrimination and prejudice. To mention biology, to confront our impairments, has been to risk the oppressors seizing on evidence that disability is 'really' about physical limitation after all."[3]

Given the huge entrenched views on disability within a medical model, one can well imagine why Mike Oliver and others have, in highlighting a social model, sought to drag people from the individual-based approach. What are needed are comprehensive views of the situation. Some have talked of a social model of impairment and of disability, in which impairment is not denied, and the debate factors in social issues such as access and employment and medical problems such as pain and chronic ill health. These do not individualize and make their situation tragic, but merely—and humanely—recognize the situation as it is. For there are many other examples within the experience of disabled people of problems not easily fitted in a social model. Sally French, who has a visual problem, writes: "Various profound social problems that I encounter as a visually impaired person, which impinge on my life far more than indecipherable notices or the lack of bleeper crossings, are more difficult to regard as entirely socially produced or amendable to social action. Such problems include my inability to recognise people . . . and not being able to read nonverbal cues or emit them correctly."

She continues:

When discussing these issues with disabled people who adhere strictly to the definition of disability as "socially imposed restriction," I am either politely reminded that I am talking about "impairment"; not "disability," or that the problems I describe have nothing to do with lack of sight, but do indeed lie "out there" in the physical and social environment; my lack or perception of this is put down to my prolonged socialization as a disabled person. Being told that my definitions are wrong . . . tends to close the discussion prematurely: my experiences are compartmentalised, with someone else being the judge of which are and which are not worthy of consideration. This gives rise to feelings of estrangement and alienation.[4]

If this is the case within the disability movement, it is almost more so for able-bodied people. To be told by an, at times, quite militant group that disability is due to social oppression can lead to tensions, and may not be the best way of reaching consensus. One person within the disability movement told me that he occasionally has to follow the more militant campaigners—"the disability terrorists"—and repair the damage done to relations between rulemakers, employers, architects, and disabled people. No one likes to be told they are wrong, that their concepts and ideas are simplistic, or that by their lack of action they are oppressing others.

As ever, Mike Oliver is aware of such a trap. I had asked him whether there was a less confrontational way? He replied that historically little progress was made until disabled people joined together and started to fight their case. Their demands, after all, were not large: "If you look at the agenda that disabled people want, they are not asking for anything different. They just want what you have got."

I remained concerned that once disabled people are seen as being part of a movement they are seen as different, and that once they asked for things from a position "outside," and when seen as not being "like us," then their legitimacy might be reduced. Should we not see them as being like able-bodied people, but with additional needs? I was arguing for an inclusive approach depending on individual respect first and foremost with the needs of disability subsequent to that.

Mike was unconvinced. "Yes, but where has the liberal position got us in the past? Those with [financial and political control] have always been the white middle class. When the transition to socialism occurs, then maybe we can all be people. My argument is that we cannot reach that state or stage with capitalism, since that requires people at the top and requires people at the bottom, and if the only way we can get to the top is by clambering over people and pushing them down, then it is a journey not worth taking."

Much, I suspect, depends on how available people in a society are to listen and how prepared to change according to the needs of minorities. From this perspective, the focus on disability and the social model makes sense. But there are also problems for disabled people if they do not accept their impairments and fail to allow public awareness of them. Jenny Morris writes, "We can insist that society disables us by its prejudice and by its failure to meet the needs created by disability, but to deny the personal experience of disability is, in the end, to collude in our oppression."[5]

If disabled people only stress the social and allow their personal impairments to remain private, then their needs as a consequence of their impairments may not be met, or may be left out of provisions. By trying too hard to externalize and socialize their disabilities, there is a risk of neglect toward their other problems.

These are complex issues, made more so by the lack of clear water between the disability and the impairment, and for the need for balance between those with different disabilities and the rest of us. Those with spinal cord injury, living from a wheelchair, may have their disability removed from the workplace by good access, adapted computers, and so on, but then such adaptation might be difficult to use for those with visual problems. Such adaptations are time consuming and costly, too. If the workplace was adapted for someone in a wheelchair, this would in turn make it difficult for a six-foot able-bodied man.

According to French, "Even if it were possible to transform the world to eliminate the disabilities of a small minority of people, would there not be a danger of disabling the rest of the population?"

Consensus or conflict? By stealth and subtle seduction, Stephen Duckworth has spent years persuading and cajoling politicians, at various levels, to the advantages of meeting the requirements of those with disabilities. While not denying their needs for financial support, for PAs and independent living, or for alterations in the built environment and public transport, he has also been chipping away at the advantages to society as a whole from the integration of disabled people, both in humane terms but also because many with disabilities have useful skills. John Hull, an academic who is blind, once told me how good he was in committee because he was less distracted by the weather outside or by the legs of the woman opposite. Stephen makes the point of how organized people with disability have to be, and how this can be of great value in the workplace.

By contrast, there is Mike Oliver, a left-wing Marxist professor of disability studies who has, in the past, quoted a Conservative Secretary of State for Health under Thatcher on the need to avoid dependency in our provisions of benefits. As ever, there may not be a single answer, and by their differing agendas, Stephen and Mike may complement each other.

I have highlighted the work of two people as exemplars of two opposing perspectives and methods. But, as ever, their apparently opposed views overlap and even coexist. In this the disability movement is no different from other political groups full of differing views and argument.

John Hockenberry, a journalist and paraplegic, expressed his experiences of the disability movement and its paradoxes thus:

You do not have to feel guilty for causing my situation. . . . You do have to feel guilty and fawning and contrite if I ever catch you using a wheelchair stall in an airport men's room. I feel as though I caused my situation and deserve to be cast from society. . . . I am a poster boy demanding a handout. . . . I have an unlimited amount of "courage" which is evident to everyone but myself and other crips. I am in denial. I have accepted my disability and have discovered within myself a sublime reservoir of truth. I can't accept my disability, and the only truth I am aware of is that my life is shit and everyone is making it worse. I am part of the disability rights movement. I am a sell out wannabe TV star media scumbag who has turned his back on other crips.

I am grateful for the Americans with Disabilities Act, which I think has heralded a new era of civil rights in this country. I think the Americans with Disabilities Act is the most useless, empty, unenforceable law of the last quarter century. . . .

I think that the disabled community is a tough, uncompromising coalition of activists. I think the disabled community is a back-biting assembly of noisy, mutually suspicious clowns who would eagerly sell out any revolution to appear on a telethon.

I'm telling you these things because I want us to share, and for you to understand my experiences and then, together, bridge the gulf between us. I want you to leave me alone.

Everything you think about me is right. Everything you think is wrong.[6]

Disability politics, like any politics, is at the mercy of individuals and ideas, movements and money. What is undeniable, however, is that through the efforts of groupings together of many disabled people, the conditions under which disabled people live and work have improved over the last thirty or so years, as they have left long-term institutional care, taken control of their lives, and live and work independently. That so much has been achieved may be commendable, but there is still a huge amount to be done to allow people with impairments to have some of the chances in life the rest of us often take for granted.

Stigma

Much of the writings within disability studies have a sociological framework, for good reason—they are trying to overcome the older "medical models" that focussed on impairment. Any notion of a Darwinian origin to stigma seemed absent. In a harsh world of natural selection, it is easy to see how physical impairment leading to disability would have been selected against (though of course difference within a population is also necessary). Then we might have developed prejudices against some forms of difference.

Oliver quotes some anthropological data suggesting that disability was not always considered a handicap, but it is not clear whether this was the exception.[7] There is, for instance, evidence that atypical faces may be related to poor health, and with a relative lessening of fitness to reproduce, which may explain their being seen as less attractive.

For Mike Oliver, such ideas were passé. "Darwin for me is a stage theorist, and I have troubles with all stage theories. I go back to Marx. I do not think the roots of our stigma are located in biological difference. I need to interpret it differently. In some cultures and some times, disabled people are not stigmatized, so we need another mechanism."

Instead he locates the origin of stigma in industrialization. As work became more regimented and needed workers to conform more to produce goods, those who could not work for whatever reason were marginalized and stigmatized. When society was more agricultural and less pressured by the need for production, disabled people may have been less stigmatized.

Such a viewpoint may strike some as unnecessarily restrictive. There are many jobs, mainly manual, unavailable to disabled people of various kinds, and this was the case before industrialization. True agrarian societies may have been more able to support physically disabled people than migratory hunting ones, but even they would have been hard for the frail. Those with facial disfigurement find prejudice and stigma all around them—unfortunately—when they have no physical impairment.[8] To deny a biological depth to stigma may not be the best way forward, even though no one would wish to argue that stigma adhered only to neo-Darwinian rules.

In support of Michael's case, there are fewer and fewer rational reasons to marginalize those with physical impairments. With white collar work and the use of computing and other devices, the range of jobs where people with spinal cord injury can compete with able-bodied people is increasing. And, as Stephen Duckworth never tires of telling potential employers, disabled people can be very good workers, because they have to be organized and resourceful, and are frequently attuned to others and their needs. They have also managed huge change in their lives, and so are well equipped to manage change at work. Both Stephen and Michael are among those trying to show this to government, to the able bodied, and, of course, to those with impairments as well.

The "big idea" moved disability from an individual impairment to the environment and to society. As we have seen, quite how to define the relationship between neurological impairment and disability has been debated within the disability movement for several years. How to best assist those with various impairments, disabilities, needs, and feelings has become a political as much as a health issue. We can only hope to air some of the issues.

The next and final two narratives give the experiences of two younger men. One became tetraplegic in his teens, the other in his late twenties. Both have been injured ten years or so. These stories may not appear so dramatic, but it is precisely by the comparative lack of disruption in their lives that one can measure their success. This is not because their injuries were less severe, or their periods in the hospital less traumatic, but because they were able to recover, indeed retain, their independence, partly because of the changes in attitude and facilities for tetraplegics they inherited and benefited from, and—perhaps more importantly—because of something within them.

VII | Continuing

16 | For What I Am

His father met me at the door. Tony was a little behind in getting up, so I sat and talked with the dog, an awesomely bright Jack Russell called Jack, until Tony came in. He was in his mid thirties, in a chair, with his arms laid out in front of him. He steered using a stick placed in front of his face, a little like Bob Dylan's harmonica.

"It was around teatime, August 26, 1992. I was on holiday in Majorca and made a mistake. It was the shallow end of a pool where I had been swimming for years. I dived in, and that was that. I have absolutely no idea how it happened. It was before happy hour, so I had not had a drink. I can't remember anything until I came around beside the pool surrounded by people. I knew instantly something very serious had happened because of the buzzing feeling.

"All my body was buzzing like mad, and I actually felt as if I was leaving myself. I know some people have this great idea that if something really serious happens they feel this, but it actually did feel like that, purely because of the buzzing. People were shouting to get an ambulance. Someone said 'Don't move,' so I didn't. Apparently, I was lying on top of the water, and someone had noticed me and fished me out. My girlfriend was in a big panic. Then the ambulance arrived and I was put into the usual neck collars and rushed into hospital.

"It was a very hazy time. I can remember lying in the bed in traction, in Majorca—fabulous hospital—smelling the suntan oil. I could see the top of the palm trees and I could hear the aircraft landing. I remember thinking to myself, 'What have you done now?' I chose the right time to do it, if there is a right time, insofar as there was a Spinal Injuries Convention taking place in Barcelona at the Guttmann Centre."

I mentioned that I had been there, presenting some work. It was immediately after the Olympics and coincided with the Special Olympics. I saw the hundred-meter final for men with visual impairment.

"So while you were in your conferences I was in traction. They flew someone from Barcelona over and he decided to fix me there and then. I had completely broken C4. I had absolutely no idea at all of the consequences of breaking your neck. As far as I was concerned, when you broke your neck you died. I'd had some perception of people in wheelchairs but, like everybody else, I thought that was a condition from birth or a sudden illness.

"I was twenty-seven, in partnership with a chap in a company that dealt in fire and flood restoration work. It was a great job, a fabulous business we had built it up over ten years. We were very happy.

"The operation took place five or six days after the injury. Then my girlfriend thought that since I would be flying back soon by air ambulance she would go before me on a scheduled flight. But then the chartered aircraft did not arrive for another three days, so I had those three days on my own, probably the most difficult time I can actually remember. I couldn't move anything. I did not, at that time, have a tracheotomy. I had a tube going straight into my mouth with pipes and things everywhere. I could speak some Spanish, but with a tube down my throat I could not speak anyway. I remember a tremendous overpowering sense of isolation. I really could have done with someone there. But we were soon flown back to England and to intensive care in Salisbury for ten days, and then I went to Odstock."

Cooking Programs

"Once back in England, the nurses in intensive care were absolutely brilliant. We had a lot of fun, even after ten days of machines venting me, and everything else, we still managed to have a bottle of champagne and a couple of gin and tonics."

A lot of fun, I thought. Tony had just lost all movement and sensation from C4 down, so that he could not move beyond a shrug of the shoulders. He was not even able to move his arms. Yet he talked of fun while still in intensive care.

"I was very lucky: The care I had from the minute it happened to today, with the entire infrastructure there for me, has been remarkable. When I came back to the old Salisbury Royal Infirmary's intensive care unit, my family was waiting for me. It was a nightmare of emotion really—for them as well as me. You are so pleased to be back with them and it makes you realize the importance of having people around you that are dear to you.

"I stayed there for a few weeks, and then the consultant from the spinal unit came down and began to give me some idea of what was going to be happening. I couldn't talk then because I had a trachy, so I mouthed my words. But he knew what I was saying. He said, 'I can't give you the absolute bottom line as yet because it's still early days, but you won't be running the hundred meters again.' I understood what he meant.

"He was a fabulous consultant. Always decorating his house and coming in with a jumper covered in bits of paint. I have a great deal of respect for the man. He came in every day. He may not have been aware of how important that was, but it was very important to me at that time. He appeared very casual but knew it all underneath.

"From there I went to the spinal unit at Odstock, three miles away, for the next fifteen months. I was there so long because I picked up a pressure mark, which eventually was the size of a table tennis ball. I had to have a skin flap and was then on bed rest for a further three months. It was six months before I got out of bed. I watched an awful lot of telly. I've never watched so many cooking programs in my life.

"I was very fortunate right from the outset. I think in my own mind I take life very much as it comes. I had no cause for anger because it was a self-inflicted accident. I never directed the anger towards myself. It was just, 'fool.'

"Initially I did not feel any sense of loss. At the time I hoped that perhaps my arm might move or the finger might move or something. I was constantly re-evaluating my situation. There were a lot of young guys in there at the time and we got on really well. I was the longest on bed rest. The guy who was in the bed beside me was only seventeen. I felt very deeply for him. He was tetraplegic. Once he started getting up, he would come over and we would talk for hours. We would talk about whether you had any more movement, whether anything was happening. Then it went on to your girlfriends, what's happening in life, what you have done in life, what work did you do. We were not really then confronting what was ahead of us."

To be so concerned about another so soon was remarkable. So unusual that the staff were concerned he was in denial and might subsequently become depressed. It never happened, though he did have one night of panic.

"When you are first in, you are positioned at the front near the nurses' desk, and then slowly, as you become less critical, you move your way down. I was in the fourth bay down. That night I woke up and went to get my buzzer, a straw which you blew to call a nurse. As I went to do it the straw came out and fell on the floor. I had a trachy in and needed suction. My chest was filling with secretions. I thought, typical, I've come all this damn way and now I am going to drown. Of course there was nothing I could do. The more I thrashed about the more I was upsetting the liquid in my chest.

"Eventually one of the guys opposite clocked it and he said, 'Tony, are you alright?' I felt like saying 'How the fuck can I answer you, I can't talk.' He said, 'Tony, just move your head if you are not all right.' So I moved, and he knew straight away there was a problem. He sounded the buzzer and the nurse came. It was pretty close.

"I had not spoken for many months. Then they weaned me from the trachy. I began to talk again, and it was incredible. You don't realize how difficult it is to communicate when you can't talk or use gestures apart from moving your mouth. Yet I still managed to converse. Quite often somebody would come along who couldn't understand what I was saying, and yet one of the guys in the wheelchairs could understand, and I would talk to him and he would tell the person. That was a really lovely experience.

"I was weaned off the breathing support gradually. This was tiring because, suddenly, the diaphragm had to do all the work. Quite a few tetraplegics get very tired and, say, reading a book find themselves asleep or that they can't concentrate. They gave some tetraplegics little oxygen masks at night. All who took part couldn't believe how awake and brighter they were."

Later he had another night he would rather forget.

"I don't quite know what happened. It was the worst night I had. It was all psychological, it must have been. I started to get very anxious. It was quite late at night, and I got more and more anxious. Maybe it was my body saying, 'Look you are not moving; you are not going to move,' and my brain thinking I want to move. I ended up in this nightmare where I thought I can't even shout, even if I shout no noise comes out because I'm ventilated. I called the nurse and said I need someone to come and sit by me—I don't know why, but I did, and the night went on and on and . . . the nurses came over quite a few times. I just had a tremendous feeling of anxiety."

Interestingly, Tony remembers this anxiety as being in his head rather than in the body or the stomach.

"The tenseness was a tremendous mental tension. It was all everything you would feel but without the butterfly bit. I felt anxiety that day like I'd never felt in my life—so if there was more feeling to come from having a body, then I did not want it that night.

"The anxiety attack went on all through the night. It was still there the next day, so I spoke to the nurse and she said there's really nothing we can do, but I'll call Nigel [the clinical psychologist]. He came to see me, by which time I was absolutely exhausted. I was anxious, but without knowing what about—that's why I couldn't get rid of it. Even if I shouted no noise came out, so I shouted as much as I liked—but it did not make any difference. I was really tired.

"So when Nigel arrived he said, 'Do you want to talk?' I said, 'No, all I want you to do is just stay there,' and I fell asleep. I woke up about an hour and a half later and he was still there. I have a lot of respect for that. He said, 'How are you feeling?' I said, 'I can't believe I had a night like that.' He said, 'Do you want to discuss it?' I said, 'I don't know what to discuss, I don't know what caused it. I haven't had a big emotional attack about what's happened.' It never happened again, so I can't really tell you why."

Dysreflexia

After six months, they put Tony on a tilting table to reintroduce him to sitting upright. Each day he was brought a little more vertical. After such a long time horizontal it was not surprising that he ran into problems.

"Soon I was very light headed as the blood drained from my head. Then I was introduced to that wonderful little thing called autonomic dysreflexia. I had been told about it, but did not know what it felt like. I was going to find out.

"One day I went vertical and everyone was saying, 'How do you feel?' I said, 'I feel like Hannibal Lecter strapped into this thing.' Then, suddenly, with a tremendous vengeance, it began. I felt some perspiration and this headache coming in really fast, and I said 'I think there is something wrong.' They saw blotchiness on my skin and someone said, 'Right. Let's get him out of there.' As I was levelled down, the dysreflexia cut in big time with perspiration, a feeling of fever, and then the headache took over everything.

"I couldn't see a thing for minutes on end [due to poor blood flow to part of the brain]. I've never had one like it, or as strong since. It was just an unbelievable experience. I did not know what to think. In fact, I couldn't think; the booming in the head was too bad. Apparently I ran the blood pressure meter off the scale. We don't know what the cause was. It wasn't the usual blocked catheter. I just know that when I lay back down again it was a good hour before I managed to really get back to any state. My hands and feet were still freezing. Apparently, if you touched my hands it was like they were in the freezer.

"I had a pill to reduce the blood pressure. Unfortunately, from then onwards I became hypersensitive. I had thirty-two attacks in seven days. You couldn't wash me, especially around my groin, because off it would go again. So in the end I said, 'Just leave me alone.'

"The headache was what I hated. It really hurt, worse than anything I had had before or since. Over the next few weeks, fortunately, it lessened."

Ten Out of Ten

"Next I learned about root pain. That suddenly reared its ugly head after a few months. One day I woke up with more buzzing. Even though I could not move or feel anything, my hands were buzzing, and my shins, feet, hands, groin, and sometimes tummy. I felt this phenomenal pain in my foot, and I thought something was wrong, so I called the nurse over. Unless something was really bad, I did not like to bother the nurses. One came over and said everything looked OK, and that I needed one of the consultants. He explained about root pain. It was very strong, tiringly strong, and would bring water to my eyes.

"It was quite upsetting, especially since I could not move to make it better or worse. I was its prisoner. It was a shooting feeling that impacts. In your hands it made you grind your teeth; it was almost like someone standing on them, especially around your nails. The double whammy was that I had pain where I could not feel: in my groin, bottom, shin, feet, and hands, always the same places. Sleep was off and on. Most of the time you are so tired from the day, tired from the pain, that you would find any way of distraction, talking to people, anything. I even watched television; things have got to be pretty bad if you start watching *Neighbours*.

"By then I was used to my environment and I drew people in. After six months in bed you need to be stimulated, so I would ask whoever was walking past for a chat. I would try and direct questions more at them than about me. They were not interested in you. I would ask, 'How's the family?' to promote talk. That would help distract me from the pain, but there were some days when it was very bad. I would pull the blanket and sheet up and try to stay as warm as possible. I became a little introverted. That's pretty much bound to happen, really.

"No drugs worked. I remember having my first pint of lager and thinking what a relief that was. I remember being on the bed and really wanting to go to the Christmas party downstairs and the sister on did not think I was ready. I said, 'There's the lift, this is a bed. Bed fits in lift, let's go.' She relented, and so I went for a few beers. It was so nice just to leave yourself for a while and be sociable, just to leave it all upstairs, leave all the pipes and tubes and noise, and watch some flashing lights and have a couple of beers. That helped the pain, but it did not mean I was going to drink every night. I knew I was either going to have to get used to it or be a fiend in some other way.

"It's very difficult because when you go out with friends, none of us wants to go harping on and moaning. It's really important that I can control the pain, so if I do go out with friends I don't let it beat me. But if it is very bad I will relax, stay indoors, and take it easy because it's the only way to do it. You do get used to it.

"There was a young guy who was a paratrooper, tough as old boots, shot at point blank range in an accident. He had terrible root pain, and I can remember zooming over to his bed in my chair and staying there while he was crying, saying to him, 'I've experienced some of that. The nurses can't give you anything, don't have anything. It's very tough, but you do eventually get used to it and you find ways of dealing with it. If it's a bad day, stay in, stay warm, don't try and do too much.' That's all you are capable of anyway.

"It was ten out of ten for months, but fortunately I don't recall giving a ten for some years now. So even if it's bad now, it's probably only a five or six. Now it's more of a consistent irritation. Losing it and leaving it behind in those intense states was heaven. It is so tiring to have that sort of pain, especially when you are trying not to show it. When I started back with the company I couldn't go in there and start talking about the pain I was feeling. I never mentioned it."

I said that Guttmann hardly ever mentioned pain. I think this was because he thought the best treatment was distraction. Certainly there was no medical treatment that worked; there still is not, on the whole.

"Things have moved on a lot since then. I don't think we should ignore it. It should be discussed and people made to realize they are not the only one. Maybe if it's shared with others it is not so bad. You really have to avoid being short with people.

"My pain can be brought on if, for instance, I haven't had a bowel action for a few days. Something is usually causing it. It's so frustrating. You don't know why you are being short with people and you can't control it. It was never within your character, and that I hated more than the pain itself. When I have bad pain, it's very important being in my bed, being secure. Then I don't have to put on a great show. I don't have to pretend it's not there"

Buzzing and Me

"But I would not want to be without some buzzing. It gives me a sense of identity in my body. I still view my body as whole; it's just motionless. I'm not a head on a bag of potatoes. I still know it's there, I still like it; I like to see it, it is still me, and I am still it, totally. I know that a lot of people are concerned because they get little pot tetraplegic bellies, and

how you see yourself aesthetically is a massive change and hugely important. But I always say at the end of the day I am motionless, but I am
still me, body and all.

"For example, wheelchairs. Lads sit together discussing what wheelchair they are going to have—the sleekest, lightest framed, super sporty
looking numbers. With electric wheelchairs it's no different. It's like buying a car, but it's actually more than that because it's part of you. But
how you perceive yourself sat in it is very important. When I am sat in
this I am very comfortable, and aesthetically I am comfortable with how
it looks and how I am in it.

"I love all the people that care for me like my family. I employ them
all myself and they are all ages. But when we are initially setting me up
in the chair, I say it is very important how I am aesthetically. I like it to
be just so. I don't want my trousers to be six inches away from my shoes.
They are fabulous with that. It's not being fussy. You do it automatically
for yourself, but I cannot, so I have to ask you to do it for me. When I
go out, you must see that I am comfortable and you are happy with how
I look. That means when I go into a meeting I don't feel compromised
by how I am dressed. I wouldn't have been before, and I sure ain't going
to be now."

Once out of bed Tony began to look around and consider his position
with others. He soon decided that so much depended on him. People
would wonder how he coped. For him it was no big deal.

"There was a guy in the Spinal Unit because he had thrown himself off
a bridge. He also had a serious mental health problem; you don't throw
yourself off a bridge for fun. One day I was in my chair by the nurses' desk
with three or four others, mainly paraplegics. He came past and, as he was
going down the corridor, someone said, 'He doesn't know how lucky he
is. He ought to be in your situation, Tony.' I said, 'Well you've missed the
point entirely. I am far, far better off than he is. He has something that you
can't see; he threw himself off a bridge.'"

Upright

I asked about being upright and how important this was. I was meaning
standing, either in a frame, or ideally, on his own. But this was not how
Tony took it.

"I love being upright. I think because I had a time, after I came out, when I had a skin mark appear, and this cost me up to three or four years on and off of bed rest, missing days out with friends, time in the summer. That cost me dearly, so the idea of lying down is unappealing, except it's nice when I am cozy in the evening or if I am tired. It's not the same having people around if you're lying in bed. You can't converse properly."

Tony's upright was being in a chair, not my upright at all. He did not even consider standing. I tried again.

"As in literally standing? No. Once I got in the chair, I wasn't thinking about the long term, I was thinking of how lovely it is to be up. Because I could not move and could not balance, there was little for the physiotherapists to do in rehabilitation. They just put a device on my neck so I could strengthen up my neck muscles. It is tiring sitting in a chair, especially with weak neck muscles. I also use my neck for all sorts of things, even to scratch my face. Everything is dropped into my belly, so even the diaphragm gets tired. Once my breathing is tired then I have had it—time to go to bed. Early days in the hospital I used to get very very tired; my stamina and strength all came later."

Being in a chair had other drawbacks too.

"I was in the chair—great—but then I found out how isolated that could be. Everyone in manual wheelchairs would go off. Even C5/C6 tetras could get about to a degree, but I couldn't. I was limited to electric wheelchairs, and most of those had hand controls, and so I was just sat there, unable to move around all day.

"They eventually found me an electric chair with a chin control. The first one was a great chair—wonderful. At long last I had motion, and it was me that was making the motion happen. I could decide when and where I was going to go, and I would go outside and down to the fields, down to the helipad, into the new hospital, exploring the world. There were regular visits to the bar, and this brought me into being part of the group. I can remember coming back from the bar and having six or seven manual wheelchairs all hanging onto the back of my chair like a big road train. We went full blast and we had some great fun."

Tony had his first outing into town.

"I had absolutely no idea what it was like to leave the confines of the hospital. I had a tremendous perception of speed in the bus. Anything over thirty miles per hour absolutely terrified me. Don't know why. Once in town, I got out, and then I suddenly realized we were all in wheelchairs and thought about peoples' perception of me. Worse, I had to challenge myself about disability. I was being wheeled towards a zebra crossing by a nurse, all wrapped up, when I saw, across the other side, somebody with a condition which made them contorted. I thought I would not want to be associated with that person. Then I could not believe my prejudice. I was so angry with myself for even contemplating that. I feel so deeply about prejudice and there was me doing exactly that. It never happened again."

Everything, All Together

Though physiotherapy could not do much, occupational therapy was helpful, and Tony learned to use a computer. He began to think about the future. But it was around this time that he and his girlfriend of seven years split up. Their house was auctioned. At the same time his business partner brought others in to do his work. Both hurt, though neither was a prolonged problem.

"The house went to auction and my girlfriend was devastated—every time she came to the Spinal Unit she cried. It was difficult for both of us, but it seemed pointless to be so upset. She had dreams of a big house with lots of bedrooms and children."

The hospital did not really know where to send Tony. He went to look at a Cheshire Home with a nurse and a community liaison officer. They were shown a room where all the inmates were building a giant octopus. The brochure for the home mentioned a lively bar; it was empty and looked completely deserted. Fortunately, the three of them had a sense of humor. Leaving in the lift they were in hysterics.

Next he looked at a nursing home, an old mansion Gainsborough had painted.

"It was amazing. I wasn't aware then that it was for the elderly mental ill. There was nobody my own age, but it was near where I wanted to be and had lots of lovely grounds where, I thought, I could disappear. I moved in and stayed for two years. It was reminiscent of *One Flew Over the Cuckoo's Nest*. I had some incredible experiences in there. There were a lot of young people working there and I think, for them, it was fun to have me there, and we all used to go out. At the top of the house there was a lady, she was ninety-odd, and going up there to have tea with her was an experience, like going back eighty years."

"I really enjoyed some of the elderly people. One of the eighty-year-old ladies used to stand in the doorway completely naked. On the first day my father arrived, in front of a beautiful sweeping staircase, he went over to ask where I was. Up went her dress. There was a lady who had been a very famous golf champion years ago. She had a massive modern art collection and a huge collection of silver. She always wore Gucci clothes and a Tiffany choker. Above her bed was a painting of a dachshund, which looked pretty rough to me, but turned out to be an original Warhol."

Once settled in, he told his business partner that he was going back to work. He needed transport and, in the end, found a London cab. He just sat in the back, but if they had stopped quickly, he would have been through the front windshield. He realized he could not return to working out on the road.

By this time he had also started a relationship. She asked him to stay with her and, like a shot, he agreed. But it was a logistical nightmare. A male friend would arrive, lift him out of the chair onto the bed, and then his girlfriend would take care of him. The friend would come back in the morning, after Tony's girlfriend had washed him and put his clothes back on, to transfer him back into the chair.

This all took its toll. He wanted to do everything in one go, and to be the same as he was before: work, girlfriend, doing everything. But it was too soon.

"This girl and I got on brilliantly. I never perceived myself as someone that someone else would take on. You can't help but feel inadequate. She would tell me the chair is academic; it's you I want to be with. But I wasn't ready. There were ridiculous things going through my mind then, like she could do so much better and how she would have a much more fruitful life, especially since she was a really attractive girl. They were all misconceptions, I think, because really the issue was whether she loved me or not, and if she did, why did I even consider those? But I did.

"Combined with everything else, I wasn't really ready, so, after eighteen months, I finished it. It was very tough. She was devastated, and I couldn't explain at the time. There was so much happening, and also I was suffering with quite a lot of pain. I couldn't explain that to anybody because I did not really want people to notice. Otherwise they might suggest I should not be doing so much. I think I was trying to prove something at work."

He knew he had been trying to prove something with his girlfriend as well. I suggested that as people get to know each other their physicality was less important.

"Yes, and in a lot of cases tetraplegic/paraplegic people end up marrying their carers. Two nurses from Odstock married people who had been in a long time. They see the person, not the disability, but it takes a lot for the person in the chair to realize that. There are underlying fears of how good you are. Your sexuality is impaired—part of sexuality is the caressing, and suddenly you can't do that. You want to be able to give, and that takes a lot of thought, a lot of talking. The talks on sexuality in the hospital say that you have sexuality and concentrate on the practical. What they can't tell you is the emotional side, and the fact that it can be very beautiful if the person is obviously consenting to those wishes for you. You have to understand each other's needs. OK, you don't get the final result at the end, but it can be just as fulfilling, important, and necessary, and you still have the same drive."

I mentioned that people who are blind may have a greater sense of tactile intimacy. They know their family, friends, and loved ones through voice, and their wives and young family through touch as well. Tony thought for some moments.

"Touch when being blind: It must be beautiful to use that sense so much. Some people find you as an individual, because of the chair and the way you are, untouchable. But all my friends do the complete opposite—they are very tactile with me. They will kiss me and some will hug me.

"I tend to ask people to hug me. My godson is seventeen now. It was difficult the first time; he did not know what to do. So I said, 'Are you going to give me a hug then?' He has been doing it ever since. There are about eight little ones I know from friends, and I adore them. They come flying in here, straight on my lap. They are not bothered. Always give me a big cuddle. They were brought up with it. Never known me any other way, and even the ones that do, they are in their twenties and they are just lovely. When I have known someone for a while I'll ask him or her to hug me."

Chair Wars

I asked what was the secret of living from a wheelchair, without any movement or sensation? Tony did not hesitate.

"Family and friends. I have a fabulous family. I've worked with my Dad—he's worked for me for many years as a carer. I didn't see a great deal of my brother before the accident, but after I saw him every single weekend. He ended up marrying one of the nurses from Odstock. My business partner was amazing.

"I just hope I can get through to people to treat me the same, love me for who I am. I am good friends still with my ex-girlfriend of seven years. She married, and the guy she married is terrific. He gives me a hug, kisses goodbye, and we get on so well. Their children are lovely. Someone asked if I was envious of him. I said not at all. I admire him, how can I be envious? I am incredibly happy for all of them as a family, and I am happy I had seven very good years.

"If you conduct yourself with a genuine sense of compassion and fairness, regardless of whether you are in a wheelchair or not, then I think you reap what you sow.

"One guy in the unit was so difficult. He was about twenty-two. His Dad was a drug runner between Spain and Morocco. He was a young rogue living in Torquay, stealing cars, robbing nightclubs, and so on. All these so-called friends he had when they went clubbing and taking drugs, where were they when he was in hospital? Once two or three people turned up, but otherwise, apart from his mother, no one.

"One day his father appeared in a big black Mercedes. Butter would not have melted in this guy's mouth. He was dapper, with a young lady on his arm. I remember talking to him. I asked if, living in Spain, he saw much of his son before the accident. He said it was very difficult, and he only came to the ward a few times. I was naughty, but I was pointing out he had come too late.

"Not surprisingly, the son was pretty difficult. One day he smashed his room up and threw his television about—not easy for someone who is tetraplegic. He even pulled his catheter out with half his bladder in it. I was in the OT department and they asked if I could have a chat with him. He just sat there laughing.

"We had an interesting tête-à-tête one day. I was in my manual chair—because we only had one electric wheelchair to share in the unit, so every other day I had the manual chair. On that day, unless I could convince someone's parents to wheel me to where I could talk to some people, I just sat and watched the world go by. Now in his time, this chap had been very violent. He came over and rammed his chair into the side of mine. Then he did it again. He said, 'Not a lot you can do about it is there?' I said everyone has his moment and left it at that.

"Two days later it was my turn for the electric chair. It weighs eighteen stone and I weigh eleven, so there was 420 pounds of weight. I knew exactly what I was going to do in this chair. I wasn't ever going to hurt him, but I would teach him a lesson. I drove up to the brand new chair his father had brought him and banged into its side. Then I reversed and did it again. I said, 'Nothing you can do about it is there? It's payback time.' I did not want to damage his chair, but I showed him that we were all in the same boat. We called it a day and he has been terrific with me ever since."

Moving On

After two years in the old people's home, he thought it time to move on. With help from his father, from friends, and from the Independent Living Foundation, he found a house nearby. It was in a pretty bad state, so they punched some walls through and made it accessible. Tony would live in his own house with a team of carers to assist.

"Another new experience, living in the community. At last I was out the clutches of those who wrapped me in cotton wool. I wasn't going to have loads of people around me, but I could choose to do what I wanted to, choose the color of my environment, invite people around for dinner. Friends and children could pop in; a massive change. I employ whom I want, when I want. It may be more expensive, but the main thing is if we are going to have a fair, unprejudiced, democracy society, then you can't lock us up.

"One of my ideal jobs would be to go from school to school explaining disability. I would really enjoy trying to break down some of the barriers. It is happening a lot more now—I see children going off to school in wheelchairs. I was lucky I was injured just as Care in the Community came in, and I was lucky to be given my own home."

Through all this he kept working. A year after he moved in, things became fairly difficult in the business because of bad debts. Out of the blue, they were approached by a company wanting to buy them. Tony and his partner agreed, once they had secured most of the jobs in their old company.

"The new MD was a good man and said, 'Your partner is going to be employed by us, what about you?' I said, 'If you are going to make a job just for me, I don't want it.' They gave me a job running the office in an administrative level and saw how I got on. It was too much. Not because of the work, but because the pressure sore kept putting me on bed rest. In the end I was compromising the sore by my determination to work. We decided I would move to credit control; I knew all the loss adjusters and they all knew me. So I took on the Southwest Region and was able to work from home. They offered to put a lift in their Bristol office, but I like working from home, so I did not pursue it. When Wales opened up I took on some work for them as well, and now I occasionally zoom over to Bristol and Cardiff for meetings, but usually I work from home, and I love it. It keeps me active and involved.

"I miss the old company and I miss working with people. But I am very fortunate that some of the staff still come to see me. At the moment this is very comfortable. I love the industry and the stories. It keeps you mentally active and alert."

Whole Again?

At the beginning of our meeting, both Tony and his father had said that nothing was off limits. So I asked about death and suicide, though his attitude to these questions was already clear in everything he said. More than that, if his words showed his love of life and creative response to the injury, then sitting with him amplified this a thousand fold. He was so animated and interested; he gestured not with arms and body but, beautifully, with his face and head movements. He was as vivid and alive a person as I have met.

Tony replied that he had once given a seminar for psychologists on living with spinal cord injury. At the end he had teased the audience that even after questions no one had asked about the big two: sex and death.

"Because I love living so much, that someone would consider suicide fills me with horror and with such a deep sadness for them. I had a transitional period, when at odd times I felt low, but never depressed. When I was in Odstock, there were always family members or an individual who was upset. I would try to spend a bit of time with them, just talking. You did not necessarily have the answers, but at least they felt better afterwards. When people were newly coming in and I was much further down the line, I could see the state of the parents, deeply upset about the future. I was quite happy sitting there, having a cup of coffee, talking them through the next few months. It was a great opportunity and a tremendously worthy job.

"There was one able-bodied guy who had tried to commit suicide, jumped off a bridge and ended up with a spinal cord injury. I spent a lot of time talking to his parents, trying to understand why someone would want to do it in the first place. The amazing thing now is that he lives in a contented fashion in his own place and goes to meetings and talks to people who suffer depression. When he had severe depression, before he jumped, people disregarded it and pushed it away. He would go into a secure unit and come out without his issues being resolved. So he thought, no one can help me—over the top, splat. Then he had a condition people could see. Suddenly people listened and were interested. He did extremely well."

What of being able bodied again? He thought carefully. "I would want to be whole again. I love what I've learned through being what I am. I've learned a great deal about people, more than I could have possibly imagined about myself, and I would like to put something bit back. Physically, I would be able to do so much more. Not because I want to play football again, although I would quite like to play rugby, perhaps. I don't think I could go back to doing a normal job, just bringing in the money. It would have to be something that helped those with disabilities."

We were all talked out. The dog was pleased, because all day he had tried to leap into Tony's lap for some affection. Tony used to take Jack for a spin on the wheelchair around the garden. Jack adored him—even though Tony could not cuddle him or stroke him at all, or even allow him close to his face. None of this mattered, for Tony's generosity of spirit and enjoyment of life were evident. I saw that, and so could Jack.

17   Finding New Things

The Medical Association of Spinal Cord Injury Professionals, or MASCIP, was meeting in Warwick, and a group of us went to encourage people to research into the treatment of chronic pain. The day started with two people with spinal cord injury giving short talks about their experiences, under the title, "What Works for Me." Nasser, who was twenty-eight and had been tetraplegic exactly half his life, was one of the speakers.

His talk was as much about the effect his injury had had on his family and on those around him as on himself. Nasser talked of how his time at university had allowed him to understand how able-bodied people view and react to impairments. He ended by saying that he required no sympathy—he had not overcome his disability. All he hoped to do was to suggest that he had taken what he could from his disability to be as independent and empowered as he could. A few months later, I went to hear more. Nasser was tanned but tired; he had returned from a holiday in Tenerife the previous day.

Nasser had gone to a big city grammar school. In the spring term, the school calendar said swimming or gym. On his first day of sport after Christmas, Nasser and his class were due to swim. Each boy was to do a two-length sprint and then see how his times improved over the term.

"We got changed and went to the pool. Over Christmas they had installed starting blocks at the shallow end, so we went up to the deep end and did two lengths' warm up. The teacher arrived and said we were starting at the shallow end. He explained that the blocks were for the swimming team and that anyone who did not know how to use them should not. We trooped down the shallow end. I was in the front, and so I went first.

"He did not tell me to dive, but the implication was there. I dived in and hit the bottom. I remember everything. I floated up on my front. I could not move anything. I felt like a mushroom, face down, staring at the bottom. My goggles had come off. My arms were floating. I could not move my neck.

"The boys thought I was joking. I was in the middle of the shallow end. The teacher was on one side and the boys the other. One boy jumped in and turned me over. I do not know how long this took. I lay there. I knew what I had done straight away. . . . I had absolutely no movement. My arms were hanging, slumped in the water. I could not move anything. There was no pain—quite the opposite, there was no feeling at all. I bobbed up and down. Ironically my mother used to say, 'Don't do that, or you'll break your neck,' when I used to swing around the stair banisters. Maybe, I thought, I have broken my neck. It was so serious it had to be something like that.

"The schoolteacher said that I had just hit my head and was in shock and that it would recover. But I knew straight away. I did not argue, but I did say in the pool that I was paralyzed. The teacher did not jump in, did not want to get his tracksuit wet. He said stay in the water, being held up by the lad.

"The other boys left for the changing room. The school nurse arrived, then a porter and the pool maintenance man. They jumped in and lifted me onto the side of the pool. They turned me over and put me in the recovery position. I don't remember panicking. I did not try to fight it, but I presume this was because I could not move. But I did try to move—it was extraordinary to see my arms and legs and to be unable to move them."

Once it was seen that he was breathing, he was picked up and carried by the porters to the teacher's office. One man had the arms and another the legs, with the nurse holding his head as best she could. At this point Nasser's neck started to hurt. He kept asking the nurse to do something about his neck; he had no way of supporting it. Once in the office he was put in a chair. He just flopped like jelly, with the nurse holding his head and a porter his body. By now the pain in his neck was almost unbearable and, presumably, had not been helped by his neck care thus far.

The ambulance was not long. He was lifted onto a narrow chair and wheeled out. He remembers going down the school drive looking up at the streetlamps.

"It was a funny experience. People are always shocked that it happened in such supervised conditions and that I was not mucking about. I did not muck about as a child. I had had private swimming lessons, was competent, and I could dive into deep water. But I had never dived into the shallow end. So the teacher had no reason to expect me to be able to do that, and neither did he say do a shallow dive, you are going into three feet of water. The alternative is that I should have realized this, and changed my dive. But I only knew one dive."

At the hospital, Nasser remembers masters around the bed and, later, his father. Most of the time he drifted in and out of consciousness. By 6 p.m. he was in a noisy ward, face down on a turning bed. A doctor came, stood by him and said, "You know what you've done don't you?" Nasser said "Yes." He still told him. "You've busted your neck." Nasser asked if there was a cure. The doctor shrugged his shoulders and walked off. For the first time, Nasser cried.

"It's funny what goes through your mind at such times. I was supposed to be going skiing with the school and I wondered how I would go. That night I should have been training for cross-country and thought I should catch up next week. There were also positives; I missed a Latin test I had not learned."

He was taken to intensive care and put into traction.

"No one ever explained to me what was going to happen. Even the consultants never explained, maybe because of my age. I was very frightened, since I had the skull traction with only a local anesthetic. I spent the night there—the most frightening and uncomfortable night of my life. I could move nothing, and was very thirsty. They would not give me a drink, and just wiped my mouth with ice cubes or with sponges. The night went on forever."

The next morning he was transferred to the nearest spinal unit, slowly, in an ambulance with a police escort. He immediately liked the atmosphere there. They replaced the four-piece traction with a two-piece and put him on a turning bed. Twenty-four hours after the accident he was in a four-bed spinal intensive care unit overlooking a marina on the coast. The pain in his neck had worsened and was, by now, unbearable.

He found he was most comfortable with his arms out at right angles, with his legs straight out below, like a crucifixion, so they shoved two dinner trays under the mattress to support his arms. After a week he developed some shoulder movement, so they put big inflatable splints on his arms with springs attached to drip stands. He moved his arms up and down for hours. Gradually his acute pain subsided.

Letters

His injury had a huge effect in the school. They had a collection: 1,500 boys were asked for fifty pence each. They bought a TV/video—he thought it was great, because he was not normally allowed to watch TV. But the effects of his injury stretched beyond the school. Councillors and MPs were involved, and within months, diving was banned in swimming pools in the area.

Though TV took up a fair amount of his time, he could not watch for long—he had to do his mail.

"Bar being dead, I cannot imagine a larger outpouring of grief. So many wrote to my parents. There were hundreds of letters, and over 90 percent of the school wrote. Many of the people from school I hardly knew. There was a huge pure emotional outpouring almost as if I had died. It was just the way they found the words to say what they felt. 'Nasser was always such a nice boy.' Or 'He was so good to have around.' I am not criticizing, but when I read or listened it was as though I was not going to be doing anything."

He realized from the letters that the injury was a long-term thing; the letters told him more than the doctors. He had a wonderful letter from Frank Williams, boss of the Grand Prix team, who is tetraplegic, and some from Manchester United and Liverpool football players. Some even dropped by. Roaul Dahl wrote, because Nasser's mother had delivered one of his daughters. The cast of *Coronation Street* wrote, and

John Thaw, the actor, wrote a lovely letter, too. Nasser wrote to him recently when Thaw was very ill himself.

Letters would take two hours per day. His mother stayed for the first week, while his father held the fort at home. Nasser's two brothers, aged eight and fifteen, needed looking after. It was an exceptionally difficult time for his family—his grandmother had been diagnosed as having terminal cancer and was in a hospice, and his mother had a slipped disc in her back and was considering a laminectomy.

When the letters died down a little, he returned to his studies. He had been due to take Maths GCSE (a national exam usually taken at fifteen or sixteen) a year early. After two weeks, a woman from the local educational authority came in, reinforcing Nasser's idea that he was not going anywhere for a while. There was some concern in the hospital that if he failed in the exam in the summer it would knock his confidence, but he had no thought of not doing it. Within a month, he had a reading stand over the bed, doing matrixes and algebra. He dictated either to the woman, or to his math teacher. It developed his memory and his skills with a personal assistant. Television soon palled.

Visitors began to arrive. His parents were always there, but soon came brothers, aunts, and friends. His form teacher drew up a rota for school friends to visit. After that, school chums arrived with regularity and precision. Nasser was pleased to see them all, but there were also times when he was grateful to be left in peace. They were forced to ask the same questions.[1]

His teacher, Peter, was a strict disciplinarian. Cards would arrive from his class with a note from Peter about how he had had to lock the boys out of the classroom again for misbehaving.

"He was a great inspiration at that time, but recently told me of how I was to him, too. When I was back out I joined the class on a visit to some docks, which was very important for me. On the way back he remembers asking me how I was feeling, and I said that 'I just have to get on with it. No cure, just get on with it.' He took strength from that and always remembered it. Recently he had to deal with his wife's death. He remembered 'No cure, make the most of it.' So through our own trials and tribulations we have helped each other."

The only time he remembers being angry was when the swimming teacher came. He stood at the bed and said, "You did not hit your head on the bottom of the pool." He thought the force of the water had done it. Nasser was very angry. Everyone else was just getting on and not trying to look back. That was the last time they spoke, though the teacher did stay on for three more years.

His grandmother was in a hospice and his mother was having traction for her neck. His father would drive to see Granny, then to see his mother in another hospital, and then see Nasser and try to eat something along the way. His brothers had to live with all this. His mother would say to people, if you want to help, cook us a meal.

"It can be harder for relatives at that stage. They do not know what you are going through. I was sort of all right, really. They were struggling to see someone go through it; I was getting the help. If the doctors were not explaining to me, then I am sure they were not explaining to my parents, either."

A Long Moment of Numbness

Nasser tried to move on many occasions. Lying in bed, unable to see his arms and legs, it was as though they did not exist, and only when he saw them was there a will to move. In fact, in addition to some movement of the shoulders (Nasser finished essentially with a C5/C6 complete level), he developed a small wiggle with the big toe on his left foot. He has some touch and temperature perception, but none of pain below the level.

"You could put a knife in and I would know you were doing something, but have no pain. In the shower I can feel something on the legs, but not temperature. The feeling is like, say, before my accident if I had had bad pins and needles and then the pain wears off. Then you are left with a moment of numbness. This is what I have."

Escape

He had thought he was busy in bed with academic work and letters, but once up in April, until his discharge in September, his time became really busy with rehabilitation and physiotherapy all day and then, in the evenings, two hours of visitors.

"First thing, the night staff would wake you and throw your clothes at you and tell you to get dressed. You were still rolling around the bed two hours later when the day staff came on at 8 a.m. I do not dress myself now. I have to get up at 6 a.m. to get to work at 8:15 as it is. I could not get dressed and then do a full day's work.

  ˋ "To function fully in society and with employment there is a point when you have to have help. Having help, are you dependent or is it about having help on your terms? As long as it is provided with dignity and on your own terms, then I would argue that this is fine. Some fight it and try to do everything on their own. I know one guy who will set the alarm at five and spend hours dressing himself, but he does not do anything when he is up. I was always adamant that I would go back to school, drive a car, go to university, do everything my friends were doing. So I accepted the help and prioritized my needs and wants."

At the spinal unit they wanted Nasser to stay a few more weeks, but he was adamant he wanted to leave in early September, in time for the new school year. He could not transfer between car and chair well, so he suggested he might return for an afternoon to learn. But it never happened. "Once you are free you are free. The best way to learn is to do it. No toilet is ever the right height out there and you just have to learn. Doing is the best education."

His accident was in January. In September he rejoined the same school year group he had left, as they all moved up a year. And he got an A in math.

Nasser came home in September. His mother came out of the hospital, having had surgery on her neck, on September 7. They moved house on the 9th; Nasser came out on the 11th and went back to school on the 14th. At school they had installed ramps and an accessible toilet, and they timetabled his lessons for the ground floor. It seemed relatively easy to put his school friends at ease. Maybe, he thinks, it is easier when younger. He had not chosen a career, so he could adapt to his new situation. Two previous ideas, the army and veterinary medicine, were clearly out. "I was glad I had it at fourteen rather than twenty-four, because I might have struggled to come to terms with it. By twenty-four, or thirty-four, you have made a life."

Initially he dictated everything or used a computer with a stick strapped to his hand. Then, at Christmas, his mother asked him to sign a few cards. He used a piece of foam, like pipe lagging, around a pen and found he could scribble. After half a dozen cards, he realized that he could write quicker than he could type. Some exams he wrote, some he dictated, with extra time allowed.

His school viewed university as being as much about having a good time and growing up as reading for a degree. They suggested he follow his interests and then, later, convert to a vocational course. He chose history at Warwick. Going to university was the first time he had been away, or been looked after by community service volunteers. He drove down a few days early, found his room, and met his assistants for the first time—two strangers who were, immediately and with no prior experience, to look after him.

Warwick was actually very good in looking after his special needs. If Nasser needed a dropped curb they would do it, if necessary closing the road for the morning. He loved the course and the study. In his final year he went to Venice for three months—a young tetraplegic in one of the least accessible places imaginable.

"I had two community service volunteers with me, and we lived in a ground floor flat. Unfortunately, with the floods, nothing happens on the ground floor. There were three steps inside the door. I studied just behind St Mark's Square. I got off the boat each morning and had to go over two bridges to get there. It was a real experience. I needed two to lift me up and down the steps. I had an English lad who had run a garden center, but the other was a slight Danish girl. They just carried me up and down. Locals thought we were mad. All the streets were cobbled and the buildings had no lifts. I did go over the Rialto once, just to say I had done it. And I went round the Doge's Palace and across the Bridge of Sighs, taking both wheels off my chair to do it."

He came back for Christmas, a little too late to apply for a further course, so he took a year off, working for a solicitor. He also had some time off for a tendon transfer that gave him greater straightening of the elbow, "useful for opening wine bottles." Then off to Nottingham Law School for a year. He had decided on law when seeing his claim for compensation taking four years or so after his injury.

He has been at the firm since, specializing in personal injury. Nasser enjoys the work and the contact with clients. He has to take witness statements, go out to see the paving stone they tripped over, arrange a doctor's opinion, and, as he does this, build up a relationship with the client. He would like to move into more work with those with spinal cord injury, not simply because he knows he would be good at the legal aspect but, of course, because he would have much more to contribute.

"With the newly injured in the hospital, the legal aspect would initially be secondary. I can wheel up and take them through the legal aspect, but also say that I was there in the bed fifteen years ago, and you will be able to drive a car, and have a job, and live independently, and have a drink with friends on a Saturday night. I could show someone they can have a life as well as helping them professionally."

Downhill Racer

When on holiday in Tenerife he was amazed by the number of people in wheelchairs there, and by how accessible and accepting hotels and restaurants were.

"Tenerife surprised me; it is so good for integrating disabled people with society. At this time of year there were so many disabled, and there were ramps and lifts and no one batted an eyelid when you turned up at breakfast in a wheelchair. It would be nice when it is no more than wearing glasses, for instance."[2]

He goes skiing every other year in northern Sweden. "I use a cart, on four skis with two levers to steer. You are six inches off the ground; sitting with knees up to chest, like a motorized go cart with a crash helmet. The ski instructors sometimes take these things down the mountain themselves because they get such a thrill from it, more than when skiing.

"The pleasure of doing it is the same as before. The first time I saw a cart I was disappointed by the way it looked, but as soon as I was on snow it was great. It is so heavy that once started it will not stop, so you have to do a driving test before. You come down fast and could wipe out kids at the bottom having a lesson. It is huge adrenalin rush. You control it with your strength. At the bottom your hands and shoulders ache. You ski with others in carts, some able bodied, some other disabled, and with people skiing normally. There is a great pleasure from controlling it with my body.

"When someone who has a limited movement, whatever it is, overcomes it, then the achievement is still there. Maybe relative to an able-bodied person the thrill is more."

I wondered if people with spinal cord injury were adrenalin junkies any more than others because such sports are beyond their reach much of the time. Nasser thought not.

"Some are active sport junkies, but the main reason is to show someone, especially newer injured—say eighteen to twenty-four months after—that they can do it. Put them in a situation they may never be in again, and may not want to be again, but show them they can do it. If you can boat across a lake, then you contemplate driving a car or doing night school. The mountain stroll, horse riding, or abseiling all allow fun and achievement, but also allow them to go back into the ordinary world, too."

He had tried horse riding and powerboats, but liked neither. Horses were too unpredictable and he was too high off the ground. I agreed. In the boat he could not balance, but at least he had had a try.[3] His present holidays are not just about skiing, any more than anyone else's is. There is the joshing between friends.

"When we go away, there are guys who are good C7s who are almost independent. Some C5s are complete and cannot feed themselves, but stick them in a cart and they can ski down a mountain. The range of dependency is quite large, but when all together we take the mickey out of each other about what we can and cannot do, as well as passing on tips."

A day on the death carts followed by a few beers must bond you together quite well.

Old Fart?

Going back to his old unit recently, Nasser saw its new buildings for the first time. Compared with the old one, the facilities were fantastic. But it was on two floors, with out patients upstairs and the gym for in patients on the floor below.

"Before everyone mixed, old and new. Those lying in bed with a pressure sore or the new ones would be there together, and out-patients would help with the tea and meals and would go out for a chip run. We learned lots from each other at different stages. When I went back there was one guy who did not want to get up and go to the gym, and the staff said OK. This surprised me. When I was in, if I had said I did not want to go to the gym, then I would have been wheeled there and put out on the floor so I was stuck and could not leave for the duration of the session. I was not allowed to just watch TV. If a consultant said you must go to gym to learn how to transfer, and the patient says well, I went down and couldn't do it, that would not be the end of it. It took me three months to learn to do it. Once in the gym is not enough.

"What the patient wants now, the patient gets. But what they want is not what they may need, or be good for them in the long term. After all, Guttmann got them out of bed and made them do things, not for him but for them.

"You need everything on one floor. When I was there last time, there was a physio session in the gym, while at same time up the other end able-bodied people were paying to use the gym for basketball. OK, it brings in money. But surely not when the spinal patients are at the other end; salt in the wounds, surely."

Nasser was at risk of sounding like an old fart, and of course knew it. But he was concerned to strike a balance between what could be achieved toward one's own independence through one's own efforts, and a realistic view of the need for aids and assistance.

"Each person needs to explore his limits physically, with his new body, as well as his mental needs for support."

He is still exploring.

"I have been in a chair fourteen years and I do not know my body. It still surprises me. Coming back from holiday yesterday, my bottom was so sore. It was only a four-hour flight, but I could not move during it. I was sure I would have a red spot but did not. But I do not know why it hurt so much. I flew to New Zealand and sat for twenty-six hours and did not have a problem at all. It annoyed me yesterday, since I was expecting something. I am constantly finding new things and new ways my body works."

On his flight from Tenerife he was in a transit van at the airport, waiting to board with four or five others who were fairly elderly. They were using airport wheelchairs to board more easily. Nasser was at the end, and the guy came over and took his arm expecting him to get up and walk.

"I thought it was funny and I said to him, 'Do you think I would be in here if I did not have to be?'[4] But I was with people who might have said the same. The assumption in airports is that people are in wheelchairs not because they cannot walk, but because they can only walk a short way. I always demand that my chair is taken to the side of the plane. The carousel damages the chair, and anyway I don't want to be sat in a small airport chair. It happened during a stopover for four hours at Singapore. The guy wanted to know why I needed my own chair and I said it was like having to wear shoes that were too small, even though it is a weak comparison."

Compensations

Nasser has managed to build his career and has supported those with spinal injury through various trusteeships and committee work. His fascination is with the balance between financial compensation for injury and the need to live life independently. He is sure, for instance, that after injuries there needs to be early release of some money as cases go through the courts.

"Some adapted vehicles cost £50,000, and are necessary to allow disabled people to go out and recover their independence. Defendants should see that, by getting claimants an adapted house or car as soon as possible, the claim is reduced the long run. The longer a person is in an unadapted house and immobile, the more chance they will remain incapable of doing anything themselves subsequently. Then, if they have not learned to bathe or shower, the judge will award a larger sum for a more complex bath. If a claimant is not going out and enjoying life, then the settlement for lack of amenity and quality of life will be greater."

He is also convinced of the need to treat people individually. "No two people are the same. It may take some longer than others; women may not want to work. It is important to allow any individual to do as much as he or she wants. A judge would never penalize a tetraplegic for not driving, or not working, or not going back to university, if it was too difficult. The sympathy of the court will be with the wheelchair person.

"To help those with spinal cord injury, I am on a career ladder. I have a mixed caseload, with mostly traffic accidents. There are some 'slippers and trippers' and a few—still—with Thalidomide with missing fingers. I am early in my career, and for the moment have to have a senior legal partner with me."

The problem, we agreed, was how to encourage people to work and become independent, without removing the safety net for those who could not.

"Maybe units have to follow up and encourage. In New Zealand, they suggested there were too many benefits to get people back to work. Here it is not the case, but nowadays it is not expected for a SCI person to work. That should be changed. I know a guy who just retired after being injured for forty years. When it happened his company just asked when he was coming back to work. There was never any suggestion that he would not work."

We returned to compensation, and the catch within. Big claims may not be settled for seven or eight years, and people may be in trouble financially until the payment. Worse than this, however, if people wait too long and hope for a huge sum, they put their lives on hold, thinking everything will be fine once the money comes. By the time it arrives, they have become dependent. Better, he thinks, to work and get out into the world.

"People have this idea that once the money is there life will start again and everything will be OK. Then they get it and realize that everything is not OK. They have had their life on hold; they have not got on with their schooling, not gone to university, not started to drive. They end up with £2M in the bank, but their lives often do not resume."

He explained that the largest part of any claim in the United Kingdom is usually for loss of earnings. Pain and suffering is only a small part of the claim for a tetraplegic, about 5 percent. You can be penalized for making an effort to advance your own life, and to an extent this is what happened to him. He was fourteen when he became unable to move below the upper arm. He did his math in the hospital, went back to school to take five more GCSEs the summer after. He finished with five As and a B, rejoined his old school year, did A levels, went to university, and became a lawyer. Along the way he passed his driving test. Nasser had no evidence of loss of earnings, and the injury had disrupted the narrative flow of his life as little as one could imagine.

If he had just given up and sat in front of the television, he would have received a much larger settlement, though he would have had a far poorer life. He has carried on not by ignoring the impairment but by downplaying the disability. "People have got to be interested in me for the person I am, not the one that I was before the injury." It has changed him, but in no way diminished him.

VIII Commentary

18 | The Dreary Ooze

The Reverend Albert Bull

In discussing the history of cosmetic and plastic surgery to the face, Sander Gilman suggested that many people have surgery not to appear beautiful but simply "to pass," to be unnoticed and accepted within a certain peer group.[1] Such passing is not an option for those with spinal cord injury. They know they will always be "that guy in the chair" to new people they meet. Not only new people, either, as one woman said to me.

"I used to go on a Saturday night, but there was never any one interesting to talk with, just drunks I went to school with who would say how sorry they were. Please go away, I'd say, and please move that cigarette away from my shoulder. I don't like making an entrance and an exit. I hate it to have a group of people lined up to say goodbye."

The chair may not simply prevent anonymity and passing, even among friends; it may also preclude a natural flow of conversation and social interaction. Sometimes with friends we might be enthusiastic and upbeat about something, and wish to make an entrance; at other times we might wish for a quieter time. The chair imposes on both by requiring the same inconveniences each and every time, flattening—or at least making more difficult—the projections of altered mood and some of the ease of conversation. In Merleau-Ponty's phrase, it imposes a style.

Much of the success of those with spinal cord injury may be viewed in re-introducing their own style, with and beyond their injury. Because a lack of standing and walking almost exemplify all disabilities, a wheelchair existence is not defined and explored for what it is, but rather for what it reveals to be absent. One irony is that for many with spinal cord injury the lack of locomotion is an inconvenience but less of a problem than pain and incontinence. Tetraplegics may lose their anonymity without others having a real understanding of their problems.

John Hockenberry's work is so rich because it shows existence in a chair positively, in terms of his attitude, in the way it gives flesh to wheelchair existence, and in the way his spirit transcends his impairment.[2] It is by reaching out to others and not being defined solely by his impairment, any more or less than anyone else is defined by their physicality, that he "passes." More, by reminding people that we are all impaired or imperfect in some way or other, Hockenberry pleads for tolerance. "All human bodies have bodies which define their existence . . . openly acknowledging limitations binds people together."[3]

The present narratives have moved from those who endure to those whose lives have been affected far less by their injury. It would be simplistic to think that we might be able to understand fully quite why these differences in response occur. There are, however, some obvious places to start, and many of these are independent of the spinal injury: chronic pain, and poor circumstances and support. In others the reasons are less clear, though there are clues. Tony, a C4 tetraplegic, was actually quite unpopular with the senior nurses on his ward because the young nurses would hang around him rather than help with the other patients. He had such an amazing social facility and interest in others that he just sucked people to him. Colin, in contrast, finds small talk, gossip, and other people difficult and so, in turn, is less approachable.

Stephen Bradshaw of the Spinal Injuries Association, himself injured, is clear that one of the most precious gifts of all is good social skills. These skills are usually present or not, but it is becoming increasingly clear that people can actually be helped with them. The British charity "Changing Faces" has been one organization leading the way in empowering those with facial disfigurement. It has shown how effective such education can be, defusing teasing and increasing confidence, as well as in educating teachers and employers.[4]

Such ideas are not wholly new. In her biography of Sir Ludwig Guttmann, Susan Goodman writes,

Guttmann found self-written reports by patients, which he encouraged, to be of enormous help in their overall treatment. These reports recorded individual reactions; patients' innate attitudes towards their incapacities, their families and society in general, freely expressed. He maintained that all his professional life he continued to learn from his patients. But he always believed that the single remark from which he learnt most—and which he never forgot or ceased to quote—was written by the Reverend Albert Bull, a paraplegic Army chaplain who had spent eighteen painful months at various hospitals before arriving at Stoke Mandeville in 1944. He wrote: "The first duty of a paraplegic is to cheer up his visitors." Guttmann felt that "This significant remark taught me and my staff how to educate the public to abandon its attitude of pity and replace it by positive and practical help in returning their paralysed fellow men and women to society."[5]

"To cheer up the visitors," as Guttmann said, there is a need to deflect pity, and this seems still the case today. But it may be this pity, and the model of spinal cord injury as tragedy, that can be so destructive and that Michael Oliver and many others are seeking to overturn. The neurological impairment, they are saying again and again, is there, OK, but do not heap on top of it social isolation, lack of access to buses, banks, buildings, and employment. For it is those social aspects of disability that are really the most distressing.

"To cheer up the visitors." Coming to a ward full of people with spinal injuries, visitors may be scared and often find it very difficult to relate to the patients, even to their husband or wife newly injured, as Kevin Hill found. Many find social interaction with a group of disabled people difficult. The patient then needs to be an expert not only in managing their own impairment, but also at putting visitors at ease, showing them that they are OK underneath. Indeed, an essential skill for a person with SCI may be this ability to reach out to and reassure the able bodied. The patient, after all, lives with his or her impairment all the time, whereas a visitor sees it occasionally. This social skill of putting others at ease with impairment is certainly a very important key to success with others and in developing rapport, as those working with facial disfigurement have found.[6]

In reacting with pity, people are also revealing their own concerns. Robert Murphy wrote of how "the paralytic's inertia is symbolic of death itself; he is life's negativity. He represents an inverse definition of wholeness; he is a living reminder of the frailty of the body."[7] From the outside, to live from a wheelchair can seem unimaginable, the ultimate tragedy and the ultimate threat to one's self and one's esteem. What if it happened to me, or my family. . . ? This may be why people working with tetraplegia on the wards do not like to get too close, and why the doctor suggested I did not ask what it was like. By showing that life goes on after paralysis, the patient can reduce these concerns. To keep the visitors happy is to say that, whatever happens, I remain human, and remain a person in relation to those around us, with all the needs and things to offer—and more—that I had before.

Stages

This is not to diminish the misery that some people feel living with tetraplegia. The factors contributing to this include pain and poor social conditions, and in addition, a model of the impairment as tragedy. It may prevent an acceptance when some tetraplegics relate their experiences of enjoyment of life and changed priorities. Mike Oliver places himself in this group, but Tony never felt a sense of loss, and Nasser adapted well and without the long coming to terms that stage theories might have predicted. John Hockenberry refuses to talk of tragedy:

I was "dealing" with nothing. . . . The future seemed like an adventure on some frontier of physical possibilities. Each problem—getting up, rolling over . . . needed a new solution. . . . Solving each problem offered a personal authorship to experience that had never before seemed possible.

To people on the outside it was all a mechanism, a trick for avoiding the cruelty that had caused my accident. To the outside, life in a wheelchair was life minus legs, dignity, dreams. It began to have meaning by adopting the code of denial, plus depression, plus anger, which equals acceptance. The dignity of human existence was restored . . . only after one denied what was happening, got angry, got depressed and then saw the light.

But from the inside trauma did not appear to need any additional meaning, it made sense on its own, and trauma did not seem quite so unusual or unexpected. Far from a digression in the stream of existence, trauma intensified experience, bringing forth elements of experience too easily clouded over by the seductive predictability of day-to-day so called "normal" life.[8]

Michael Oliver's thought was that only a minority of people go through stages in coming to terms with their new existence and with their injury. For him such stages serve the medical staff and people around the injured person as much as anyone. "That there are periods of mourning and denial, of anger and then restoration allows others to move on from the impairment and after a while put it behind them and expect the patient to as well."[9]

Instead it is a more lifelong process of adjusting to changed circumstances. A recent study of women aging with spinal cord injury found some people who felt the same: "People always ask me if you adjust. . . . I find it's an adjustment every time you make a major change in your life. As a disabled student, I coped. Then there was another adjustment when I went into the workforce. When I got married and had a child, there was more adjustment. Now it's adjusting to age. . . . It's always a process of adjustment—for most people that's life isn't it? But adjusting to trauma that's something in addition."[10]

Such adaptations are neither universal nor necessarily easy; for some, a period of mourning and depression may be unavoidable. In her interviews with women after spinal injury, Jenny Morris found that many struggled to find a balance between a need to be brave—largely for others—and the need to come to terms with their injury: "I tried to express my grief, but was met with a total lack of response." "The staff expected you to have a smile on your face the whole time."

The message was "be strong" for the patients, but also to spare the nurses and doctors. "The emotional side was rather suffocated. Everyone kept saying how strong I was. . . . It would have been good to have been encouraged to have had a good scream and a cry." "I often felt I was acting a role and keeping visitors at ease." "You could not talk to the staff emotionally." "In our isolated sense of grief the only source of comfort were other newly injured people, who 'were just as scared as me.'"[11]

What these differing responses are pleading for is for a service sensitive to the feelings and needs of individual people as they respond to their own injuries, and to a service that dares to ask what it is like for each person. As we have seen, again and again, the spinal cord damage may be very similar in two people, but their responses and needs for medical and psychosocial support may be vastly different.

Forgetting

Although people with spinal cord injury can discuss the differences in their lives and in the relations with their bodies that their injury has imposed, with the passing of time they become more and more used to their new bodies and their new ways of being—so much so that many people said that this was their normal now. This, of itself, is remarkable.

The absence of sensation and movement, paradoxically, makes the body more phenomenologically present and needful of attention. Remember Colin relating how vigilant he was after surgery. "Fortunately, because I have as much sensation as I have, I don't have to think, because my body tells me. When I had the first cystoscopy they gave me a spinal anaesthetic which completely numbed the body from the waist down. I found that a very difficult situation. I was totally unaware, had lost all spatial awareness of my lower body. I am constantly analyzing what I am doing. If something does not happen as before, I am always trying to think why that should have been the case and what I can do to correct it."

Others also told of how attentive they had to be to small and often inconsistent clues about their bodies. Yet despite this new relationship and attention to themselves, this became their normal, at times indistinguishable to our normal.

Graham related, "Now I can almost kid myself that I can feel something when I sit in a chair, even though I know I cannot. It feels exactly the same sitting in a chair now to before I was injured. It can't, but it does. My mind tells me so. My mind makes me think I am like you over there. It learns what is the norm for this body. It tells me there is nothing wrong, so I feel comfortable and correct. Remember, I have been longer disabled than abled. In a relatively short time things become a norm. You almost forget how it was before."

There is an element of forgetting and other elements of filling in of sensation, or its visual capture, as we have discussed. But beyond this there is also a suggestion that the brain—in part consciously but in part without effort or attention—moves the person to a state where their situation is "normalized" and restored, as best it can be. This is close to Goldstein's ideas of how a disordered organism, and by extension an individual, regains a state of order.[12] He wrote of performances being modified to reduce the deficits, but later of a "capacity for a shifting of attitude." Many people whose narratives we have explored have shown such a shift as they have explored what is possible, bringing together their remaining capacities and capabilities to make a whole, their whole. This is not to mean that their impairment is no longer seen as such or is reduced, but rather that, from what remains, they explore and construct a personality and a selfhood that becomes their normal.

I Don't Want You to Imagine Being Me

I had begun by wishing, and maybe daring, to ask what it was like to be someone else. As Robert Murphy has observed, "Nobody has ever asked me what it is like to be a paraplegic—and now a quadriplegic—for this would violate all the rules of middle-class etiquette."[13]

Such a process of "truly understanding what is in the mind of another," to paraphrase Hockenberry, might be termed empathy; Natalie Depraz and Evan Thompson have examined the process.[14] For these two philosophers empathy is not an experience by which we attempt to understand another by observing their behavior and situation with reference to our own experience. Rather, through empathy, we experience another person as a unified whole, as *their* whole.

They suggest several kinds of empathy. There is a passive association of my lived body with that of the other person as we grasp another's body as being like our own. At one level, to see another person in action is to begin to imitate their actions. There is recent abundant evidence of such imitative neural activity within our brains.[15] In a second type, there is an imaginative transposal of myself to the place of the other person—in other words, I try to imagine what it might be like to be the other person from the perspective of that other.

Kay Toombs[16] has written on the problems of achieving such empathy with people whose physicality is so different to one's own. Her interest is in medical education and its need to understand both the bodily dysfunction and the lived experience of illness, the meaning of the disruption in the context of a particular person's life situation, in order for medicine to be humanely grounded.[17] How possible is this when faced with neurological impairments so far from normal experience? Toombs suggests it begins to be possible if one engages in two processes. Observation may allow some information, but to know the experience and feelings of the other, then one must also attend to their narrative, expressed freely and in depth, which she terms "empathetic listening." Just as a medical history details the impact of the disease on the body, so the clinical narrative, a patient's story, conveys the impact of the illness on the person. She suggests, for instance, that to consider multiple sclerosis as being to do with demyelination of the central nervous system captures nothing of the lived experience of the illness. Both scientific and personal information are necessary.

For Toombs it is through clinical narratives that one can glimpse what it is like to be another, and begin to understand what it is like to have impairments beyond our experience. Then if one is to try to grasp another's experience, one has to take their narrative and use a process of imagination to attempt to see the world through the eyes of that person. This is not the same as "putting oneself in another's shoes." Such a projection may actually hinder understanding, because you are still you but in another situation. Toombs pleads for medical education—and indeed, the education of all health care professionals—to allow, in parallel with the learning of disease process and treatment, a development of the imaginative faculties so that people may not be afraid to look into what it is like to be another. Without this the experience and existence of the person with the impairment is forever beyond others. This is a humane injunction, but also necessary for appropriate care of an individual with a chronic illness.

There remains the question as to how far one can actually imagine oneself into another's life and another's body. And not all agree with such an approach to disability and impairment. For Michael Oliver this focus on the neurological impairment, rather than the social disability, is dubious, because he views his problem from a social perspective. Mike could not imagine being without spinal injury, "because it is not going to happen." Others had been injured so long that it was normal for them. If these people with experience of two bodies cannot remember or imagine their pre-injury embodiment, then how deeply and completely might I imagine what it is like to have spinal injury?

I put this to Mike, who replied, "But I don't want you to. Why should you want to? If you need to understand my needs, ask me. I don't want you to try to understand my needs and then meet them because then you might misunderstand my needs. That is what Leonard Cheshire did.[18] He tried to understand disabled people's needs; he understood in his own particular way and stuck 70,000 disabled people effectively in prisons [homes for the disabled in the UK]. Thank you."

I protested that at the time Cheshire might have salvaged a number of people's lives, even though he did it by "imprisoning" them in large homes and communities. If, at the time, people's needs had been truly understood that would not have happened.

"I see where you are coming from. I left that behind in the early '70s when I got political, when we were trying to build a movement. For the first ten years of my life as a disabled person, the only disabled people I knew were spinal cord injury or from sports. When we were trying to build a sort of coalition across impairments I started meeting blind people and deaf people. We spent the first couple of years trying to imagine what it would be like to be someone else. I would say to a blind person, 'Cor, I am glad I am not blind.' And they would say, 'I would rather be blind than be in a wheelchair like you.' We realized there was intellectual work to be done, but it was not about trying to understand how we felt about each other, because where would not get us anywhere. It was about trying to understand why we all had crappy lives.

"I don't see myself as a person with a disability. Black people don't want to be seen as people with a different colored skin, women as people with a different genital arrangement. You have to find ways of recognizing, valuing, and respecting difference rather than ignoring it. I don't want you to understand what it is like to have no control over bladder or bowel. I want you to understand that I need a job, to use the same public spaces and facilities as you, that I need a decent education and a house with a front door I own, and to control who comes in. I want you to understand those things. I don't need you to understand that I sit in this wheelchair from the neck down without feeling anything, and what it feels like, because I don't know what it feels like to have a period. In order to be sensitive to it, I don't need to know about it."

He is not arguing against a need to understand, but that this should move away from the personal to the effects of socially originating disability. In this he is echoing Stephen Duckworth's friend, Simon Brissenden, who wrote, "In order to understand disability as an experience, as a lived thing, we need much more than the medical 'facts,' however necessary these are in determining medication. The problem comes when they [medical staff] determine not only the form of treatment (if treatment is appropriate), but also the form of life for the person who happens to be disabled."[19]

The whole picture has moved from a phenomenological account of living without movement and sensation to one that includes the social problems encountered as a consequence.

"The experience of spinal injury, therefore, cannot be understood in terms of purely internal psychological or interpersonal processes, but requires a whole range of other material factors such as housing, finance, employment, the built environment and family circumstances to be taken into account. Further all these material factors can and will change over time . . . given the experience of disability a temporal dimension."[20]

Few could disagree with this. In fact, such a social or ecological perspective must be as much part of any account of living with spinal cord injury, and of any empathetic approach to another, as descriptions of the problems with sensation, continence, or movement. I have explored these matters from a training in clinical medicine and in neuroscience. But to encompass and understand, I have been pulled from medicine to wider considerations, of the built environment, of access and employment and politics. Without access to the world and without a chance of employment if wanted, a person's experience and life after spinal cord injury can be as impoverished as by the impairment.

By denying access or independence, society can make people with various impairments feel ostracized and worthless, with loss of self-esteem. Many have pointed out the importance of our social being in our perception of self. According to Robert Murphy,

human behaviour derives its organisation and content from the interaction of biological drives with culture. It is better to talk of the human condition than human nature, since our nature lies around us as much as within us. In disability biology has less to teach us than social anthropology. . . .

There can be no irreducible human nature free of society's imprint, so, too, can there be no human existence in total isolation. Alienation from others is thus a deprivation of social being. This loss of self, however, is inherent in the social isolation of paralytics, who have furthermore become separated from their bodies by neural damage, and from their former identities by society.[21]

Mike Oliver might suggest that society and the model of impairment as tragedy robbed people of identity. Only by grouping together and discovering shared experiences did the disabled regain it.

Returning to Kay Toombs' imaginative transposal, it may actually be easier for able-bodied people to relate to the social problems of spinal cord injury than to imagine life without sensation, movement, or continence. Most of us, after all, have been excluded from something at one time or another, whether a theatre or restaurant, or been unsuccessful at a job interview. No one would argue that the scale of such rejection is similar to that of people with spinal cord injury, but it does seem plausible that empathy with the disability may be easier than with the impairment. But, despite the eloquence and force of Mike Oliver's argument, it seems unproven that empathy with the social disability without consideration of the underlying neurological impairment is sufficient. In contrast, some neurological empathy seems necessary, for reasons we will consider later.

Knackered

Those of us who do not die young know that the chances are that we will suffer a period of ill health before we do die later, in "old age." Most people suffer their spinal cord injuries when relatively young, a time of risk taking and of presumed immortality, leaving them with much of their lives ahead. Care for those with spinal cord injury has had to come to term with the fact that, whereas thirty years ago or so those surviving were nearly all young, now there are increasing numbers of older tetraplegics. Indeed, there may now be two causes for this increase: men who have lived with it since their twenties and thirties, and women who become injured later in their lives.[22, 23] There is also evidence that old age itself may come earlier with tetraplegia, just as Colin and David suggested. Zarb and Oliver asked a sample of more than a hundred people who had lived with chronic impairments for many years, some of whom had spinal cord injury, for their experiences of living with impairments for decades.[24]

They found accelerated deterioration in a number of physical areas: breathing and diaphragm function, arthritis,[25] as well as the "normal" late problems associated with spinal cord injury—osteoporosis, renal and bladder problems, and the development of cysts, or syrinx (swellings in the spinal cord that could raise the effective level of the injury and remove vital hand or arm function). Among women there were also concerns about menopause and other gynecological problems.[26-29] With age, the margins for error were reduced; people simply become increasingly worn out, in their joints, bowels, bladder, bones, and even lungs, which have years of underinflation, and heart, which may not have been exercised hard for years. Muscular and skeletal joint pain is a particular problem, as joints not designed for years of transfers wear out.

A study talking with women who had lived with their spinal cord injury for a mean of twelve years and who were from thirty-five to seventy years old, found both similar and additional problems.[30] Because women are less likely to be married after spinal cord injury than men, more women live alone. Women are less likely to be employed, or to drive, and are more frequently depressed. Some have suggested that to be female and disabled is a double disadvantage. To be old may be a triple jeopardy.[31]

If all these physical matters are understandable, more perplexing is the reported widespread loss of volition. People start to feel more and more fatigued. Dressing, bathing, working, or being social are hard work in a wheelchair; with age they become all the harder as what was previously possible just becomes too much. Many have lived their lives at max, and then with old age that max declines alarmingly: "My major disability is a lack of energy—will power just isn't enough any more."

"We are always tired, so after twenty years—you're just knackered."[32]

"I'm at an aging point in only my early forties. . . . "I've got to go either into a retirement living situation or a very small place because I can't cope."[33]

With these increasing physical and volitional problems come social concerns. Living independently can become increasingly difficult, either alone or if their spouses are their PAs, because they too can become less able. For some these and the other problems may be the reason why expectations of life satisfaction decline after thirty years or so. As ever, it is difficult to generalize, because others describe an increased and profound sense of inner strength and acceptance as they age, and even suggest that their injuries have allowed them greater self-exploration and spirituality: "Now I am older I understand myself better, my limitations . . . a certain self-analysis . . . you can apply to how you cope with your body and its limitations."[34]

Some in a Canadian study suggested that once old with spinal cord injury, people know the worst is over, and that they have come to terms with their disability long before others affected only as they age. But the majority did have concerns about loss of independence, finance, and declining health superimposed on their impairment. They also felt strongly that the health care system had not really caught up with the emerging and increasing needs of those with spinal cord injury who, for the first time, were entering old age. If this is the situation in socially advantaged Canada, it is likely to be all the more so elsewhere.

Looking Forward

If these matters are of concern and worry for those with spinal cord injury, then contemporary research into spinal cord regeneration might allow more optimism than ever before. Christopher Reeve has placed himself publicly at the forefront of fundraising, giving it a public and human face. Yet among those I spoke to, there were reservations. Reeve's very public pronouncements about the pace of research and of recovery were not shared.

Tony told me, "I don't know about the Christopher Reeve idea, that I will recover, is the right way. If that works for him, then I wish him all the best. What I tend to like to look at more is what's going to better my life here and now. I don't have the finances for devices, or hordes of physios. If you have a belief and he is following that belief, then great. I don't know whether it's necessarily to say I will walk in five years. I admire Christopher Reeve in many, many ways. I think he has brought a great profile to the whole thing, but I might have just kept that five-year bit to myself."

In *Forward*, the magazine of the Spinal Injuries Association, there have been quite heated exchanges on the matter recently among those with spinal injuries. The underlying concerns were as much about being reconciled to one's life as it is, and having that way of life accepted, as about the possibilities for cure. The letters also reveal the passionate nature of the debate.

Christopher Reeve is high profile and normal rules do not apply, so he does not see all the problems. . . . From my viewpoint he has swapped superstardom for new role of victim and super cripple. Nothing has helped those who live now. . . . He is unrealistic in hope of a cure but because of his position his words take on power. . . . His promises of a cure suggest that it is wheelchair users, not society, that need to change. Pinning hopes on a cure is no way to live a life. You need a good quality of life now.[35]

Others were more sympathetic and suggested that Reeve had not shied away from being a role model. One listed the problems in waiting for a cure: "One might not live a full life now, it might create false hopes, from a social perspective the quest for cure might reinforce negative stereotypes that disability is abnormal and, lastly, if a cure was 'around the corner,' then what incentive was there to give full civil rights to those 8.5 million disabled in the UK now?"

Opinion was divided as to whether one should think of a cure or get on with it. One man wrote, "I was quite pleased to realize that we now had a champion who would work to break down the barriers that we still face. Now I fear he has, willingly or otherwise, allowed his feelings to be hijacked by the mass media, which is more interested in headlines, 'I will walk again in five years, says crippled Superman.'" Another suggested that "I can live now and hope for research and help with bowel bladder, sex, arm movement, sensation, pressure sores, root pain. The sooner you accept there is a place for both approaches, the better." This correspondent pointed out that Reeve had also set up programs to help now through Quality of Life schemes.

A woman, paraplegic since radiotherapy, was more enthusiastic. "We would have been dead but for research, and want to feel this is still going on. Christopher Reeve has decided that this is the cause he wishes to champion, and I don't think he should be criticized for doing so. I am glad the film world has not shunned him now he is disabled, but has sat up and listened. Life must always have hope."

From the outside it is difficult to see Christopher Reeve, whose level of spinal cord injury only allows limited independent breathing and little movement (at least initially), and not think that anyone in that position would seek an improvement in their impairment. Even a few centimeters of functioning cord would allow breathing and use of the arms.

Michael Oliver has long been critical of charities promising cure and that, in order to fund raise, have painted the grimmest picture, reinforcing in people's minds the tragic view of the impairment. He has even previously argued that "the aim of research should not be to make the legless normal, whatever that may mean, but to create a social environment where to be legless is irrelevant."[36] In this present debate, between those with spinal cord injury rather than academics and politicians, he was more cautious. "Twenty years is a long time to claim a cure is just round the corner. A more realistic position is that the cure is a long-term goal and, if and when it is discovered, there will still be battles to be fought to ensure reasonable access to it."

Live for today, and if a cure comes along, then all to the good. Research in the regeneration of nerve cells in spinal cord injury may not allow a tetraplegic to walk, but if it lowered the level of injury to allow a high tetraplegic to use her hands, then it may provide a major improvement for that individual. For someone requiring artificial ventilation, with an indwelling tracheotomy and all the anxieties of relying on a machine, the alteration in their level by a few centimeters might allow independence of breathing. These hopes, at least, might be noncontentious.

Reeve himself is aware of the ambivalence within the spinal cord injured community and has responded in a dignified and measured way. "Some tell me that there is no point in searching for a cure: others say that they are happy with life the way it is and don't want to be cured. It's difficult for me to understand their point of view, but I completely respect those individuals as long as they don't try to interfere with progress."[37]

Research must and will go on, but it should not diminish the equally valid need for social provisions now.[38] Underlying this debate is the nature of adapting to one's injury. Some have suggested that one has to accept that one's spinal injury is permanent before beginning to be fully reconciled to it. A health care worker in spinal injury told me that she did not think anyone was ever fully reconciled. As we have seen, for many it is a continuous process of adapting, each day to each thing. For some people the hope that one day they may be cured keeps them going, even if they may think this unlikely; for others, such an attitude prevents them from getting on with things as they are. There is no single way of living with tetraplegia, just as there is no single way of living for any of us.

Anyone who places himself in the public eye, as Reeve has done, with such an injury and who has been made into its exemplar by the press, knows that they can never please all the people all the time. Fame never comes on one's own terms. But some words of Nietzsche come to mind. In a series of aphorisms about what makes one heroic, he suggested, "to approach at the same time one's highest suffering and one's highest hope."[39]

Here and Now

Perhaps research will significantly alleviate the impairments of those with injuries, though any new treatment may be expensive and so might be rationed. It is likely also to be most effective in the most recently affected. But there are improvements needed here and now. The individual narratives given above have highlighted several issues. Perhaps the most pressing and most difficult concerns are chronic pain and continence. These are easily highlighted but less easily treated. Chronic pain, as we have seen again and again, can wreck someone's life more than paralysis and remains a major challenge. Fortunately, it has moved up the list of priorities in spinal cord injury research, with, for instance, a recent book on classification and treatment from the International Association for the Study of Pain.[40] In face-to-face interviews, the misery of incontinence was less evident, but these problems are much to the fore in continuing medical care.

From the narratives and from a small experiment by Paul Kennedy (see below), a need for prompt and continuing access to specialist units, throughout life, was also highlighted. In many countries specialist care units for those with spinal cord injury are now the norm. Yet these units may see themselves as caring for the acutely injured, or be forced to see themselves in this way by their financial managers. Continuing care of those with spinal cord injury over their whole lives, for their physical problems and their emotional support, should be the aim.

Many of the other concerns have been about the need to reduce the disability associated with spinal cord injury, whether by improving access to work, by better psychosocial support and a reduction in the perception of injury as tragedy, or by more accessibility to the general environment. Individuals such as Nasser, Graham, and Ian also suggested that those with spinal cord injury are best placed to help others with the same problems. The organizations of users groups that have developed over the last few decades allow people with spinal injury to meet and talk with others and enable them to learn more about their impairment and developments in living with it (see appendix for websites).

It must always be born in mind that people prepared to give a narrative of their life to an almost complete stranger might not be typical of the entire population of those with spinal cord injury. The larger published samples, however, are broadly in agreement. Pentland et al.'s study[41] found that many older people bemoaned the lack of help with psychosocial and emotional adjustment at the time of their injury. Some were quite bitter about this. Many, for instance, agreed that they learned most from their peers: "Getting to talk to people . . . going through the same things or are in your age group . . . is remarkable. It really, really helps me."

Often, as with Graham, the best of times was during rehab as an inpatient. Several people felt isolated and forgotten within their community. Pentland et al. made suggestions that included regular peer support groups and early and continuing support for psychological, relationship, and sexual issues. In this they are recognizing that, far from being a single event, spinal cord injury requires adjustment over the whole of one's life. Though some aspects of improved care would be expensive, the provision of better peer and psychological support for the injured and their families would not be costly. User group organisations, such as the Spinal Injuries Association of the United Kingdom, already do a huge amount. Perhaps we need to facilitate help by those adjusted to their spinal cord injury for those with more recent impairments. The formers' experience is, after all, hard won.

The Whole Certainty

Reeve described his being with spinal injury as being like a child again because he became completely dependent on others once more. Yet Stephen Duckworth, also tetraplegic, talked of how he would always offer to help with the washing up. How might this difference in perception be possible?

Gallagher makes a distinction between a sense of agency and a sense of ownership.[42] The former is the sense that I am the one who is causing or generating an action, for instance causing something to move, or who is generating a thought. The sense of ownership is the sense that I am the one undergoing the experience, that it is my body moving (whether or not the movement is initiated by me or another person or machine). In discussing functional electrical stimulation induced movements with Deborah and Julie, I tried to tease out the different feelings of control and ownership of movement with these different implants.

Because of the care they have to give to bladder, skin, and to spasms, tetraplegics continue to have a sense of embodiment, but this moves from being one primarily concerned with movement and gesture and sensation to one concerned to interpret odd sensations and feelings to aspects of embodied existence that previously were little thought about—continence and skin care, for instance.[43] Despite this, for most people their legs were still their legs, whether felt or not. Even so it seems likely that the relationship between self and body does change. Merleau-Ponty wrote that "I observe objects, but not my own body."[44] In that the normal relations between sensation and body, and between agency and movement, alter, tetraplegics may be said to observe their own bodies in a way others do not. Merleau-Ponty considered the relationships between self and thought, and body and action, further as he developed his ideas of an embodied existence.

Consciousness projects itself into the physical world and has a body . . . [it] is in the first place not a matter of "I think that" but of "I can." . . . Consciousness is being-towards-the-thing through the intermediary of the body. . . . The body is the general medium for having a world. . . . My love, hatred and will are not certain as mere thoughts about loving, hating and willing: on the contrary the whole certainty of these thoughts is owed to that of the acts of love, hatred and will of which I am quite sure because I perform them . . . I make my reality and find myself only in the act. . . . It is not because I think I am, that I am. The whole certainty of love, hatred or will is that I perform them.[45]

Many with tetraplegia are unable to act on the world in the same way as before, with profound consequences for their sense of being. Samuel Beckett wrote that "You do what you are, you do a fraction of what you are, you suffer a dreary ooze of your being into doing."[46] Those with spinal cord injury might be expected to have to negotiate such a dreary ooze each day.

Yet David, for one, suggested that the playwright was mistaken. "I think he got it the wrong way around. Yes, there are other ways of being than just doing, and probably the more creative you are the better. For me, though, I think it helps to explain my self-perception and self-image by saying that the key is doing into being—the opposite of Beckett. Dragging more out of my head into my body, spreading my physicality throughout my body, gives me the possibility of physically doing things. Being into Doing—I don't think that's right. I think the things that I do make me who I am. That need to express myself physically in certain things that lead me from the doing of things into being a person."

Similarly, Graham and then Tony realized the importance of breaking out from thought and intention to action. "Me is the mental side. I am what I think, rather than I am what I do. I release my thoughts into speech or writing or anything else, rather than into any other movement. It is still doing, but less doing. It is more intellectual, but that is one reason why I enjoy cycling, because it is a raw physical release. Before I did not realize how badly I needed it."

"They eventually found me an electric chair with a chin control—wonderful. At long last I had motion and it was me that was making the motion happen. I could decide when and where I was going to go and I would go outside and down to the fields, down to the helipad, into the new hospital, exploring the world."

Yet others talked of their doing things with little or no movement at all. This is precisely where personal assistants are so important. When Stephen talked of doing the washing up, he did not do it physically, but by asking his PA to do it he gained a sense of agency and ownership of action for himself of the task. A good PA, by acting and doing when the tetraplegic asks and in a manner satisfactory for them, can relinquish his or her own agency and give it to the tetraplegic, so allowing the tetraplegic a real sense of acting in and on the world. Tetraplegics agree that being able to order actions when and exactly how they want is crucial. To paraphrase Merleau-Ponty, "Consciousness can be a being-toward-the-thing through the intermediary of my body and that of my PA. . . . My body and that of my PA are the general media for having a world."

A PA may perform many movements, but not all. Talking with a tetraplegic one cannot help be aware of their rich vocabulary of gesture, with the arms, through movement of the chair, and in head movement, as well as through facial expression. Gesture—embodied expression—finds outlet wherever it can. And of course in love and sexuality, the personal is expressed individually and creatively despite the injury. To paraphrase once more, "The whole certainties of love, hatred, or will are still performed *but differently.*"

The Vacuum Cleaner Bag Needs Emptying

This is not to say that such relationships all proceed smoothly. A tie between an employer who is immobile and a PA who does many physical tasks for that person under their absolute direction is itself extraordinary, and may attract both good people and some more dubious sorts. Graham, it will be remembered, has had some problems in finding the right person, though others, like David, view each new PA as an opportunity. Dave Morris wrote of his first PA in terms of how he took control for the first time since his injury: "Independent living changes the usual presumption that 'crips are passive and dependent.' Living is about independence, control, spontaneity, and personal development. Why should the fact that I need somebody to wipe my bum deny my aspirations?"[47]

For the first seven years after his injury, his parents cared for him; then he was in an institution where his physical life was "standardized, routinized, pigeonholed, organized, planned." He emerged from this as "a fully fledged 'severely handicapped' crip . . . in many ways, the most striking being my retarded clothes sense. My suitcases, which filled the back of the St John's Ambulance driving me to university, bulged with neatly labelled, easy fit, Velcro-fastened crimplene creations . . . trousers too large, baggy Y-fronts. I was eighteen . . . I believed I needed to wear those things."

He applied to the one university that would take him and provide PAs. "The only person who had the same place down five times on his university application form." With an easy-going PA, for Dave the transition from dependency to spontaneity just happened. He is quite clear how important the relationship is: "It reverberates in every corner of one's life. It shares intimacy, it oversees success and failure. It is an interaction that is virtually unique. By its very nature it is physical and breaches strong social taboos. It is a relationship that is under constant flux: mutating as individual replaces individual. I have developed many short-term relationships. Each one of these . . . is fully rounded and individual, capturing a period, a space, a moment. . . ."

"Sometimes some small element within me resents having to go through the anxiety of building a relationship with a new PA. When I think about it carefully, however, the stress is vital. It is a bonding process, communication across a vast expanse of difference. Somehow I have known that my autonomy and control is directly caught up in the quality of relationship I have with those individuals providing personal assistance."

That distance between employer and PA needs to be right. Beverly Ashton writes,

Over the years I've caused myself a lot of difficulty by listening to, worrying about and taking on the life problems of PAs. I now know, without a shadow of doubt, that the best response when somebody tearfully spills out some terrible problem, is to say "Oh dear! I'm so sorry. That must be awful . . . but could you look to see whether the vacuum cleaner bag needs emptying."

In the past I have been repeatedly involved in really desperate things, marital violence, partner infidelity, teenage pregnancy right down to the death of beloved pets. I find it difficult to feign lack of interest, because I'm fascinated. These are real life soap operas. However, getting involved kills the "employer/PA relationship" stone dead.[48]

With a PA in attendance there can be problems going to the cinema, or in an intimate dinner, as the competing needs for assistance and for privacy are balanced. One woman, Ruth Bailey, now asks her PA to wait outside the cinema with a book. To manage meals out was even worse:

I can remember feeling full of despair that I would never again experience intimate dinners with friends where we talked about really personal stuff. I felt I would lose my sense of being an individual, that I was becoming one of a couple yet the partner was a PA whom I had no particular knowledge of, or feelings for, and vice versa. I am still at the stage of feeling quite uneasy about chatting away to a friend and ignoring the person sitting next to me, cutting up my food, holding my drink, or whatever.[49]

In the United Kingdom there other issues as well. It could be difficult if a PA was black, and one tetraplegic had a friendship ruined with someone who could not understand why a black person was doing all the menial work. One gay tetraplegic had a problem when his equally gay PA was flirting in a gay bar when he should have been working for him. Another was told she could not bring a heterosexual PA to a gay conference. There may also be ethical judgments to be made. What if the tetraplegic wanted to smoke dope; should a PA roll the spliff? What if it was heroin, or if his employer, devoid of the ability to act himself, wanted to take his own life? There are difficult lines to be drawn here. If a person lacks independent action, and if society is happy for someone else to provide it, then how should we set limits to a person's independence of volition and action?

No Decisions About Us Without Us

With the rise of independent living and of groups of people with various impairments to advance their rights and needs, came a realization that "experts," rather than helping, could be part of the problem. Well-meaning medical people continued to see only tragedy, with users being unfit to control their own care. In contrast, "the disabled" wanted to take control of their lives and have mainstream education and work. These were predicated on the "big idea" that Mike Oliver has already discussed. Physical impairment was not seen as "a personal tragedy deserving of sympathy, welfare, and charity." Disability was instead "the disadvantage or restriction of ability caused by a contemporary social organization which takes little or no account of people who have physical impairments and thus excludes them from participation in the mainstream of social activities." Ken Davis[50] suggests these statements and insights revolutionized disabled people's self image and allowed them to take pride in themselves as "whole beings, impairments, wheelchairs, braces, crutches, warts and all."[51]

Merleau-Ponty wrote that "the body is our medium for having a world," suggesting that it is through the physical body that we interact with and are involved with the world and with others. The big idea turns this upside down. We all need a world, a physical environment, with which our bodies can interact and so express themselves. Disability is no longer solely within the body, but also outside it. A world with inaccessible transport and buildings excludes many from any meaning within it. Unfortunately, many worlds remain beyond physically impaired people. For despite the rise of PAs, of independent living, and disability movements, there are many battles still to be won.

At a recent meeting of the United Kingdom association of spinal cord injury professionals, Paul Kennedy played a sneaky trick. He asked each group to go away and decide its five top priorities for spinal cord injured people. Each group was a different section—doctors, nurses, social workers, even people with spinal injury, "the users."

The occupational therapists' priorities were funding for adaptations, accommodation, treatment for spasms, access issues, and discrimination. The psychologists' were better post-discharge services, reduced stigma and better environment, and better communication between users and pain management. Doctors plumbed for continence and pain relief, followed by access issues and those issues to do with the human spirit and self-esteem. Lastly, the users' wish list was for full and equal opportunities and a developed Disability Discrimination Act, continence and pain relief, open access to spinal units, and finally that those people with spinal cord injury should make the decisions. "No decisions about us without us." In looking for differing perspectives among different health care workers and users, Kennedy had shown the range of issues still unresolved.

Another area still questioned is how much those with disability require the able bodied as their advocates? For many with impairments the lessons of the past thirty years are that real change requires them to take matters into their own hands and make demands. Equally for the able bodied, often those with the resources, before response comes understanding, and the fuller this can be then the deeper any subsequent involvement will be. To understand and be empathetic—with the consequences of the neurological impairment as well as the disability—is to explore these issues in one's own mind—to have one's own sense of agency for the idea—after which one is more likely to be helpful than if confronted with demands. Empathy then seems not simply a liberal luxury, but rather a part of the necessary process of personal involvement in political and social change.

Christopher Reeve, discussing the political process in relation to medical research, writes, "It is impossible to legislate compassion, yet that is what is needed most, the majority of legislators who support . . . research have an emotional connection to the issue. . . . Now we have to reach out to [those] not directly affected by disease or disability. We have to ask them to do something much more difficult, but something which will make all the difference: just imagine what it is like to be somebody else."[52]

A Task for Gods

Throughout these discussions there has been a balance between the impairment and the disability, between the social and the personal. To live with tetraplegia means to consider and explore a new relation to one's body; to go out into the world requires an exploration of access. At one level interventions try to alter the balance for those with spinal cord injury so that their "thoughts and sense of being alive are not driven back into the brain," to paraphrase Murphy, but rather are expressed in both speech and action.

Both Julie and Deborah wanted the choice whether to use their machines or not, whether to stand or not. Stephen Duckworth, in the end, said that all any of us have are time and choice. Choice here is actually close to freedom, for we all need the freedom to choose, without that choice being limited and made less spontaneous by a neurological impairment, or by an inaccessible environment.

Merleau-Ponty suggested that "freedom is doing. . . . Once my actions cease to be mine, I shall never recover them, and if I lose my hold on the world it will never be restored to me."[53] In this, in relation to spinal cord injury, as we have seen, he is fortunately now wrong. Among the aims of those helping those with spinal cord injury are to return action to them, to increase choice, spontaneity, and freedom, and to increase the potential decisions available, whether to work or not, to live independently or not, or to go out or stay at home. This is to an extent what medical support, PAs, independent living associations, and social legislation are for.

Yet there still seems to be another dimension, for even all these factors do not completely explain why some with spinal cord injury do so well and others do not, why some endure and some enjoy, as we have seen. There seem to be factors beyond both the social dimension and the neurological impairment, important though those are. Those who do well seem to be able to let go of their past in order to explore and adjust to their new lives.

Recently I attended a conference on imagination, where I gave a paper on spinal cord injury. I took a convenient definition of imagination, "the experience of sensory and or motor sequences which are independent of peripheral sensory or motor information." I spoke of early hallucinations of erroneous leg position after injury, of late phantom pain, and of the ability that people with spinal cord injury have to imagine movements, even years later, normally, as far as brain scanning can determine. I thought I would be criticized for avoiding the main issue, but was surprised that at the conference—of philosophers mainly—no one spoke of the more recent and now widest use of the term imagination to mean the creative or inventive powers within us.

Steve Mithen, an archaeologist, considered the various species of nonhuman primates in our evolutionary past.[54] Some had well-developed technical intelligence and were good hunters or toolmakers. Others might have greater abilities at socialization or a more highly developed memory. He suggests that the development of man from these early species was not initially due to the evolution of greater intelligence, but to the joining up of these various types, or modules, of cognition within our brains.[55] With such "cognitive fluidity," our ancestors were able to relate and integrate information, say about technical intelligence (thinking about objects to be manipulated) with social intelligence (thinking about people), so that the modern mind could think about a consideration of people, for example, "as objects to be manipulated."

Mithen suggests that this cross module integration was a crucial factor in our emergence, along with language and self-awareness. Cognitive fluidity allowed the development of art, with knowledge of natural history (of, say, a hoof print), combined with the technical intelligence to make an artifact and the social need to communicate intention, all harnessed to create images with symbolic meaning. This fluidity also allowed connections between objects and experiences in various modules for the development of metaphor and analogy. These two devices, he suggests, are important tools for thought and are used extensively and creatively in art and, indeed, in science. Seeing connections between apparently disparate observations and thoughts is important in both. He cites Richard Dawkins for his description of natural selection as a "blind watchmaker." Symbolism, cognitive fluidity, and metaphor may therefore define the modern mind and underpin the development of a creative imagination.

To return to spinal cord injury, with freedom and choice comes an attitude or disposition toward the world, toward others, and toward our own situation. The ability to explore a life without movement or sensation, to rebuild social relationships, to cope with incontinence, to let go of one's past and, for example, to rediscover sexual relationship without orgasm and without penetration, all require a huge reinvention. Nasser once said to me, "People have got to be interested in me for the person I am, not the one that I was before the injury." Perhaps to transcend spinal cord injury, as have many in this work, requires a creative and imaginative adaptation as one's life is rediscovered and reinvented. This imaginative capacity, which may have evolved from cognitive fluidity and allowed thought experiments and theory of mind predictions of social interactions, seems crucial in order to explore and adapt to physical change.

Just as Toombs pleaded for education to develop the imagination of medical workers, so it seems as important for those with tetraplegia. This sort of imagination and openness seems a key, perhaps *the* key, to successful living with spinal injury. Graham showed this both before and after his illness. In fact, it was this attitude as much as anything else that determined when he was head up in the world. Nasser showed the same when he said that each person must explore his limits physically and his mental needs. He is still exploring. "I have been in a chair fourteen years and I do not know my body. It still surprises me. . . . I am constantly finding new things." John Hockenberry showed the same openness and willingness to explore: "Far from being a blank wall of misery, my body now presented an intriguing puzzle of great depth and texture. To rediscover my changed body was to explore the idea of the body and its relationship to the mind in a way no night class, self-help book, or therapist could. My body may have been capable of less, but virtually all of what it could do was suddenly charged with meaning. . . .

"From the beginning disability taught that life could be reinvented. In fact such an outlook was required. The physical dimensions of life could be created, like poetry. . . . To have invented a way to move about without legs was to invent walking . . . a task reserved for gods and to perform it was deeply satisfying. None of that was apparent to the people who stared. To them, I was just in a wheelchair. To me, I was inventing a new life."[56]

If such a creative imagination is important for those with an injury, a question is whether this can be released or encouraged, to find out if people can be helped to see and enjoy those parts of their life that remain and those parts that develop subsequently. Arguably, by questioning talk of medical tragedy and passivity, and by extending his range of possible experiences in a constructive and creative way, Michael Oliver is showing such creativity. By immediately turning to look at the effects of his injury on his family, Nasser showed such an imagination, and by reaching out to others after their injuries so too, in their different ways, did Colin and Ian. Such a creative imagination is not fictional, deluding, or recursive, but rather a view of the world that is open, transcendent, and disposed toward enjoyment and enrichment, wherever it can be found. To paraphrase Wittgenstein on humor, it is not a mood but a way of looking at the world.[57]

Such an imaginative process is not simply needed in extremis, though then it is stretched and tested. We all have aspects of our lives that are routine and so can become dull. It is through this imagination and creativity that we search out new ways of looking at and enjoying the familiar; to enjoy the everyday as new and fascinating is one of the greatest of gifts. In this Murphy, despite his severe reflections on his own "descent in quadriplegia," agrees: "The paralytic is, quite literally, a prisoner of the flesh, but most humans are convicts of sorts . . . the paralytic—and all of us—will find freedom within the contours of the mind and in the transports of the imagination."[58]

Julie Hill, who has explored her paraplegia and restored her life after her injury beautifully, asked for increased choice with the LARSI system, and for the chance to fulfil a dream: "Using the implant, I will stand up from my wheelchair and hold onto the crutches I need for balance . . . the Hill family—all four of us—will link hands and make footprints in the usual thin spattering of snow."[59]

And may she do so but, lest it be forgotten, there is also an aesthetic to the wheelchair she would leave behind for that walk, if we can only see it. John Hockenberry described it, as he was going down Michigan Avenue one day:

It had been a long day. I was tired and I stopped worrying about speed and pedestrians: a dreamy dissolve . . . the walking people became moving posts in a slalom course . . . the territory between the bodies became an ether, a river of space into which I could glide. . . . Gravity pushed the chair ahead, and with the smoothness of curves on a lathe, I carved a trajectory around the pedestrians. The space between pedestrians became my space, and the whole scene unfolded as a postulate: Can this be done? Can the staccato pedestrian rhythms blend with the reedy line of effortless rolling descent? Wheel jazz.

When the fear of collision vanished, I ceased to look like a piano rolling down a hill. The chair and legs joined for all to see in an unsolicited statement of grace.[60]

Later, he had an encounter with real snow:

It took years in a wheelchair before I could be truly amazed by what it could do, and what I could do with it. On a winter night in Chicago, after a light snow, I rolled across a clean stretch of pavement and felt the smooth frictionless glide of the icy surface. I made a tight turn and chanced to look around. . . . The street-light cast soft icicle rainbows. . . . I saw two beautiful lines etched in the snow. They began in parallel and curved, then they crossed in an effortless knot at the place where [I] turned to look back. My chair had made those lines. . . . It was the first time I dared to believe that a wheelchair could make something, or even be associated with something, so beautiful.[61]

We need to encourage those with spinal cord injury to use their imagination to find what beauty, enjoyment, and contentment that they can, whether it is in a paraplegic dancing in his chair or in the cooler grace of a tetraplegic's gesture. The rest of us need to use our own imaginations and to look on without prejudice.

Appendix: Useful Websites

There are a large number of sites dedicated to user groups and health care professionals within those interested in living with spinal cord injury. With the development of links, giving an exhaustive list here seemed unnecessary. Below is a short list of those I thought most useful. The first two are possibly the widest ranging. Though primarily support groups for those with spinal cord injury, they both have extensive links to other sites.

National Spinal Cord Association (USA): ‹www.spinalcord.org›.
This has comprehensive information about all aspects of spinal cord injury, with sections on resource centers, topics (from activities of daily living to ventilators and work), publications, etc.

Spinal Injuries Association (UK): ‹www.spinal.co.uk›.
This is comprehensive, with chat rooms, advice on vacations, universities, etc. It also has good links, grouped according to American links (via <www.makoa.org/sci.htm>), British links, support, research, fact sheets, rehabilitation, newsletters and articles, books (with a link to Amazon.com), bulletin boards, chat rooms, and treatment centers.

International Spinal Research Trust: ‹www.spinal-research.org›.
Dedicated to research into cure.

Christopher Reeve Paralysis Foundation: ‹www.christopherreeve.org›.

Focussing on research, but also involved with issues related to living with spinal cord injury, quality of life, and advocacy.

Christopher and Dana Reeve Paralysis Resource Center: ‹www.paralyis.org›.

An information center for people living with paralysis and for their carers.

American Spinal Injuries Association: ‹www.asia-spinalinjury.org›.

For health care workers and patients and their families.

American Paraplegia Society: ‹www.apssci.org›

Primarily to improve the quality of medical care.

Notes

Chapter 1

1. Cole, J. D., Illis, L. S., and Sedgwick, E. M. 1987. "Pain Produced by Spinal Cord Stimulation in a Patient with Allodynia and Pseudotabes." *J. Neurol. Neurosurg. Psychiat.* 50, 1083–1084.

2. Cole, J. D., Illis, L. S. and Sedgwick, E. M. 1991. "Intractable Central Pain in Spinal Cord Injury is Not Relieved by Spinal Cord Stimulation." *Paraplegia* 29, 167–172.

3. Murphy, R. 1987. *The Body Silent.* New York: Henry Holt, p. 90.

4. Merleau-Ponty, M. 1964. *The Primacy of Perception.* Illinois: Northwestern University Press, p. 146.

5. Sacks, O. 1985. *The Man Who Mistook His Wife for a Hat.* London: Duckworth, pp. 42–52.

6. Cole, J. 1995. *Pride and a Daily Marathon.* Cambridge, MA: The MIT Press.

7. By will, in this context, I mean the action of choosing to do something, the attitude of the mind directed with conscious intention to (and which normally issues immediately in) some action, physical or mental.

8. Murphy 1987, p. 78.

9. See Treede, R.-D., and Cole, J. D. 1993. "Dissociated Secondary Hyperalgesia in a Subject with a Large Fibre Sensory Neuropathy." *Pain,* 53, 169–174.

A friend and colleague devised a contrastingly pleasant experiment. His thesis was that when people bathe and shower they are not simply cleaning themselves but grooming in a wider and altogether subtler way. So he persuaded a group of female models to shower and wash while a camera recorded their movements and time spent washing various areas of their bodies. My friend's unenviable task was to go through the tapes.

10. Is pain ever really remembered?

11. Frank, A. W. 1991. *At the Will of the Body*. Boston: Houghton Mifflin, pp. 29–30.

12. Murphy 1987, p. 75.

13. Reeve, C. 1998. *Still Me*. New York: Random House.

14. Cole 1995.

15. Goodman, S. 1986. Spirit of Stoke Mandeville: The Story of Sir Ludwig Guttmann. London: Collins, p. 96.

16. Goodman 1986.

17. Stover, S. L., DeLisa, J. A., and Whiteneck, G. G. 1995. *Spinal Cord Injury: Clinical Outcomes from the Model Systems*. Gaithersburg, MD: Aspen Publishers.

Chapter 2

1. Sir Ludwig Guttmann, founder and director of the Spinal Centre Stoke Mandeville Hospital.

2. Goodman 1986, p. 129.

3. This has been poorly recognized and understood. But any neurological illness is tiring to live with, even when little or no physical activity is required. To sustain a life under difficult circumstances seems to require an almost physical energy that, especially if prolonged, is a strain.

4. In the UK, parish councils are the smallest tier of local government and often a joke. Mine, I thought, despite my wife's best efforts, was in charge of 100 meters of footpath and four street lamps.

5. Wittgenstein, L. 1980. *Remarks on the Philosophy of Psychology*. Oxford: Blackwell, p. 31e.

6. Astronauts talk of the pleasure and relaxation that comes from living in "zero g." One even said she was homesick for space when she returned to earth.

7. Merleau-Ponty, M. 1962. *The Phenomenology of Perception*. London: Routledge; New Jersey: The Humanities Press, p. 184.

8. Robert Murphy wrote of "one man never going out and no one ever visiting, even his children's friends . . . not only the others, there is a balance between the falling back into ourselves and a need to reach out. . . . Amongst the disabled the inward pull becomes compelling, often irresistible." Murphy 1987, p. 93.

9. New boys indeed, historically. Guttmann suggests that during the First World War, survival was a few weeks to months for 47–65 percent, and that 80 percent were dead within three years. This may have been the case during the Second World War, too. Remember that these figures would have been for paraplegics and tetraplegics together—tetras would have fared the worse by far. Goodman, S 1986 p. 98.

10. In the UK, homes for the "young disabled" take the under 65s.

11. Murphy 1987, p. 18.

Chapter 3

1. Many tetraplegics have expansive use of their arms and shoulder in gesture of which they are hardly aware. Language seems to need embodied expression and will use whatever parts that move.

Interestingly, when Christopher Reeve recovered some movement of his left index finger, it was first seen associated with gesture rather than when he was making a conscious effort to move it.

Chapter 4

1. Murphy 1987, p. 27.

2. Gallagher, S. 1986. "Lived Body and Environment." *Research in Phenomenology* 16, 139–170.

3. Leder, D. 1990. *The Absent Body*. Chicago: University of Chicago Press.

4. Merleau-Ponty, 1962, p. 91.

5. Frith, C. D., Blakemore, S-J., and Wolpert, D. M. 2000. "Abnormalities in the Awareness and Control of Action." *Phil. Trans. R. Soc. B* 355, 1771–1788.

6. Reeve 1998.

7. Murphy 1987, p. 90.

8. Humphrey, N. 2002. *The Mind Made Flesh*. Oxford: Oxford University Press.

9. Murphy 1987, p. 90–91.

10. Ibid., p. 92.

11. LeDoux, J. 1998. *The Emotional Brain*. New York: Simon and Schuster.

12. Damasio, A. 1999. *The Feeling of What Happens*. New York: Random House, pp. 289–290.

13. The question of more than academic interest here is whether emotional experience might be dulled in those with tetraplegia because the flow of information between brain and body is so disrupted. As both authors suggest, however, this is a gross over-simplification. If one needs the body to experience emotion, then those with spinal cord injury maintain normal facial feedback and also have feedback, via the vagus nerve originating just above the spinal cord, which carries information from the viscera to the brain. Hormones and peptides also flow between brain and body.

It is also the case that people with a spinal cord injury, for the most part, have already learned much about emotional experience before their accident. Last, the releasers and contexts for emotion are often within a rich social relatedness, and these are still available.

Recently Ronan O'Carroll and Nigel North have assessed the abilities of people with tetraplegia to perform two tests that they presumed depended on sensory feedback from the body. In one, the Iowa Gambling task, it was assumed that success requires an element of gut feeling—from the body via sensory nerves. In the second, they were asked about their abilities to identify and describe feelings and to distinguish feelings and bodily sensations of emotional arousal, an alexithymia test. In both tests the tetraplegic group was inseparable from the control group. They concluded that spinal cord injury did not have an effect on identifying feelings or using them during gambling. They did mention that feedback from the body could have arisen from the vagus and other cranial nerves and via hormones. North, N. and O'Carroll, R. E. 2001. "Decision Making in Patients with Spinal Cord Damage: Afferent Feedback and the Somatic Marker Hypothesis." *Neuropsychologia* 39, 521–524. O'Carroll, R., Ayling, R. O'Reilly, M., and North, N. 2003 "Alexithymia and Sense of Coherence in Patients With Total Spinal Cord Transection." *Psychosom. Med.* 65, 151–155.

14. Murphy 1987, p. 87.

15. Ibid.

16. Ibid., p. 76.

17. Ibid., p. 93.

18. He also told me that he had, at last, installed a hoist to help him with transfers between bath and chair. We had argued about this with more force at the time than I implied before. Since then he has also retired early, to enjoy the cricket and much more, I hope.

19. Murphy 1987, p. 90.

20. "Humour is not a mood but a way of looking at the world." Monk, R. 1990. "Ludwig Wittgenstein." London: Cape, p. 59.

21. Beckett, S. 1958. *Happy Days*. New York: Grove Press.

22. Beckett, S. 1957. *Murphy*. New York: Grove Press, p. 2.

23. Beckett, S. 1958. *The Unnamable*. New York: Grove Press, p. 148.

24. Kapusinski, R. 2001. *The Shadow of the Sun: My African Life*. New York: Knopf; London: Allen Lane/Penguin Press, p. 138.

Chapter 5

1. Cole, J. 1998. *About Face*. Cambridge, MA: The MIT Press.

2. This was shown to be due to an inappropriate response to anti-diuretic hormone.

3. Rowe, D. 1983. *Depression: The Way Out of Your Prison*. London: Routledge. Quotes are from pp. 2–8 and 45.

4. Most sensation is conducted through the main peripheral nerves and hence the spinal cord. But some sensation may reach the brain through a more tortuous pathway, either through the vagus, a cranial nerve that supplies the viscera

of the chest and abdomen, or through the parasympathetic system, which is involved in automatic functions such as regulation of temperature and blood pressure. It is also the case that few spinal cord injuries are absolutely complete. David, with some sensation, may have some slight cord conduction.

5. The pain often felt is projected below the level of the injury but may be originating above it, analogous to phantom limb pain. That David could feel nothing if the skin was injured and yet had pain in the same area is compatible with this. Ironically, the pain he may use to feel connected is a symptom of his disconnectness.

6. Cole, 1998, p. 118ff.

Chapter 6

1. The pump is placed next to the spinal cord, in the epidural space, so that it delivers the maximum amount of drug to the affected cord. If given by mouth such a dose would cause too many side effects.

2. In one sex guide for people with spinal cord injury there are suggestions for making love in a chair, with the final sentence being to remember to put the brakes on the chair first.

3. A BBC Radio program on disability, where the title mocks the way in which people talk to the carers of people who are disabled rather than to them directly.

Chapter 7

1. Some even say that they can spot which spinal treatment center a person has been to, such is the effect of their rehabilitation and treatment on their subsequent lives.

2. One good guide to independent living for those with spinal cord injury is Sian Vasey, ed., 1999, *The Rough Guide to Managing Personal Assistants*. London: National Council for Independent Living.

3. Not just the person with the pain, either. One wife of someone with a spinal cord injury and severe pain told me that she thought it would have been better both for her and for him if he had died at the time of the injury.

The medical provision for spinal cord injury is focussed on acute care and then moves to rehabilitation. People are discharged into the community not because spinal centers do not want to look after them, but because they are so stretched, in the United Kingdom at least, caring for the "acutes." Yet people with spinal cord injury actually require extra care throughout much of their lives.

Later difficulties include hormonal problems, including high calcium, which may reflect lack of physical activity and relative bone resorption, osteoporosis, renal stones, pressure sores, recurrent urinary infections, and kidney problems. Later, serious illnesses frequently appear: septicaemia, pulmonary and circulation diseases, pneumonia, and urinary infections once more. Though the acute spinal cord break can occur within less than a second, its medical consequences continue for the rest of the person's life.

The long-term outcome for those with spinal injury is related to the level of injury and the age when it occurred. After the first year there is an 18-year survival chance overall of 75 percent, compared with 93 percent controls. A person with a high tetraplegia at twenty-five years of age has a life expectancy 44 percent of normal (see Stover et al. 1995).

4. Nepomuceno, C., Fine, P., Richards, J., et al., 1979. "Pain in Patients with Spinal Cord Injury." *Arch. Phys. Med. Rehabil.* 60, 605–609.

5. Stormer, S., Gerner, H., and Gruninger, W. 1997. "Chronic Pain/Dysaesthesia in Spinal Cord Injury Patients: Results of a Multicentre Study. *Spinal Cord 35*, 446–455.

6. Rose, M., Robinson, J., Ells, J., and Cole, J. D., 1988. "Pain Following Spinal Cord Injury: Results from a Postal Survey. *Pain 34*, 101–102.

7. Rintala, D., Loubser, P., Castro, J. et al. 1998. "Chronic Pain in a Community-based Sample of Men with Spinal Cord Injury: Prevalence, Severity and Relationship with Impairment, Disability, Handicap, and Subjective Well-being." *Arch. Phys. Med. Rehabil.* 79, 604–614.

8. For recent reviews of pain, see Putzke, J. D. and Richards, J. S. 2000. "The Impact of Pain in Spinal Cord Injury: A Case Control Study." *Rehabil. Psychol.* 45, 386–401 and Burchiel, K. L., and Yezierski, R. P., eds., 2002. "Spinal Cord Injury Pain: Assessment, Mechanisms, Management." *Progress in Pain Research and Management*, vol. 23. Seattle: International Association for the Study of Pain Press.

9. Scarry, E. 1985. *The Body in Pain.* Oxford: Oxford University Press.

10. Murphy 1987, p. 55.

11. Stover, DeLisa, and Whiteneck 1995.

12. Kennedy P., Rogers, B., Speer, S., and Frankel, H. 1999. "SCI and Attempted Suicide: A Retrospective Review." *Spinal Cord 37*, 847–852.

13. Morris, J. 1991. *Pride Against Prejudice.* London: The Women's Press. See chapter 2, "Lives not Worth Living."

14. Thompson, E. 2001. "Between Ourselves." *J. Conscious. Stud.* 8, 5–7, 197–314.

15. Depraz, N. 2001. "The Husserlian Theory of Intersubjectivity as Alterity." *J. Conscious. Stud.* 8, 5–7, 169–178.

16. In this situation we might also ask if we should go beyond the person's immediate experience and be informed by our knowledge of how others have felt at a given time in a given situation and then gone on to feel later.

17. Sacks 1985.

18. Stensman R. 1985. "Severely Mobility-Disabled People Assess the Quality of Their Lives." *Scand. J. Rehabil. Med.* 17, 87–99.

19. Stensman R. 1994. "Adjustment to Traumatic Spinal Cord Injury. A Longitudinal Study of Self-reported Quality of Life." *Paraplegia 32*, 416–422.

20. This repeated and long-term follow up is important, as it may be doubted whether people would answer a questionnaire truthfully while in a busy out-patient department.

21. Whiteneck et al., quoted in Stover et al., 1995.

22. One doctor told me that in his opinion, one-third of people do well after spinal cord injury whatever happens, one-third do badly whatever, and one-third may be helped by medical and psychosocial support.

23. Manns P. J., and Chad K. E. 2001. "Components of Quality of Life for Persons with a Quadriplegic and Paraplegic Spinal Cord Injury." *Qual. Health* Res., 11, 795–811.

Chapter 8

1. Hill, J. 2000. *Footprints in the Snow*. London: Macmillan.

2. A common perceptual disorientation.

3. The quotes in italics are from Julie's book, with her permission.

4. Normally we stand and walk without fatigue because the nervous system turns on and off muscle fibers within a given muscle sequentially, so guarding them against fatigue by rotation. FES is too crude a stimulus to allow this. In addition, muscle fiber type changes with disuse, making the fibers themselves less resistant to fatigue.

5. When Tony Tromans first mentioned the LARSI project to me in a corridor some years before, my first reaction was that it could not work, because the anatomy was against it. Any given nerve root supplies muscles with several actions that are usually antagonistic for a given movement. We did not evolve a nervous system with a single nerve root per movement. The problem may be insoluble for standing and walking. There is no pleasure in having made such a prediction.

6. Julie was not making her muscles work but was made to feel tired by the electrical stimulation of her muscles leading, one presumes, to release of chemicals from them, which led to the feeling of fatigue as they made their way to the brain. Normally, of course, tiredness is a combination of peripheral muscle fatigue and a central feeling of tiredness having made so much mental effort.

7. It was interesting that when she had the broken leg, which she could not feel, it affected her sense of self none the less. "I was amazed at how disabled I felt when I broke my leg. It made me remember my vulnerability again, since I have breezed the last ten years—and then the deep vein thrombosis and leg and I felt that my vulnerability had slapped me in the face again." It took some months to recover her normal out-going and confident self.

8. Though one can have little idea what, if anything, dreams mean, the experience of those with spinal cord injury, though disparate, perhaps reveals something of the effect of their injuries. Most people do not appear to dream of themselves with an impairment. In their samples of 205 women (Morris 1989), and of 22 people with spinal injury (Stensman 1994), most people moved around in their dreams fairly normally. But Stensman noted one young woman who took her wheelchair on her back in case she got into difficulties. He describes a number of women in whom spinal injury was present in their dreams. One dreamed of

being a marathon runner: "I often dream I am running free in the fields." Another said that it was wonderful to go to sleep because in her dreams she walked and ran. The most common dream was of walking but still having a problem, either heavy legs or where there was a chair present in the background. One woman said that "I can usually walk in my dreams, but the dreaded chair is lurking round somewhere." She could stand up and walk about, but once she sits she became paralyzed again. Another had the ultimate revenge. In her dreams, everyone but her was disabled. Morris J., ed. 1989. *Able Lives: Women's Experience of Paralysis*. London: The Women's Press. Stensman 1994.

Chapter 9

1. The spinal cord in cross section has a peripheral arc through which the fibers pass conducting up and down the cord, and a more central greyer area where the cell bodies for movement at that level are found. The sensory pathways for touch are posterior, and for movement and temperature more anterior. It is therefore possible to have some preservation of light touch but not temperature and movement if the spinal damage is anterior, which seemed to be the case for Deborah.

2. Information on the Freehand System can be found at The NeuroControl Corporation, 833 Rockside Road, Valley View, Ohio, 44125, USA. 001 216 912 0101. See also, Hobby, J., Taylor, P. N., and Esnouf, J. 2001. "Restoration of Tetraplegic Hand Function by Use of the NeuroControl Freehand System." *J. Hand Surg.* 26B, 459–464; and Keith, M. W. et al., 1996. "Tendon Transfers and Functional Electrical Stimulation for Restoration of Hand Function in Spinal Cord Injury." *J. Hand Surg.* 21A, 89–99.

3. The delay was due to technical problems. The team had to wait for new implants to be made.

4. Charles Bell made this point in his first description of movement and position sense:

I called this consciousness of muscular exertion the sixth sense. When a blind man stands upright, by what means is it that he maintains the erect position? It is obvious that he has a sense by which he knows the inclination of the body . . . . a sense of the degree of exertion in his muscular frame. . . . We stand by so fine an exercise of this power, and the muscles are from habit so directed with so much precision that we do not know how we stand. But if we attempt to walk on a narrow ledge we become subject to apprehension; the actions of the muscles are magnified and demonstrative. (Sir Charles Bell 1833. *The Hand: Its Mechanism and Endowments as Evincing Design*. London: Pickering. Reprinted by The Pilgrims Press, Brentwood, Essex, 1979).

5. The week after I met Deborah, she actually had the other side done.

6. In fact, through a series of functional brain imaging experiments it has been shown that when asked to imagine moving parts of their bodies that are paralyzed, people with quite high spinal cord injuries—and several years after the event—can still activate similar areas of brain to control subjects. Possibly their

brains have not forgotten how to move. Shoham, S., Halgren, E., Maynard, E. M., and Normann, R. A., 2001. "Motor-cortical Activity in Tetraplegics." *Nature* 413, 793.

7. Deborah's electrodes are on her finger flexors and extensors and thumb flexor, extensor, abductor, and adductor (which allow all the usual thumb movements in four directions). Wrist extension is under voluntary control but was strengthened by a tendon transfer in the forearm of an elbow flexion muscle (brachialradialis) to a wrist extension muscle (ECRB). The system therefore locks the position of her hand, rather than the wrist. The actions are complicated, however, because with finger flexion there will be a tendency for the wrist also to flex, which has to be resisted by a voluntary effort. With the buzzing and flexing of fingers, and focus on the shoulder, it is not surprising if Deborah cannot attend to all that she needs to do. I am very grateful to Paul Taylor for explaining the exact connections of the Freehand System to me.

8. The Freehand is set so that slow movement of the shoulders will not release the handgrip, but a short, sharp shrug does.

9. This distinction between a movement and its goal is a way of talking about the focus of movement used by Wolfgang Prinz and his colleagues at the Max Planck Institute in Munich, though of course Deborah did not know how perspicacious she was. Recently this group has been investigating just such a way of improving motor control by learning to focus on the goal of a complicated movement rather than on the means (and muscles) required to do it. Mechsner, F., Kerzel, D., Knoblich, G., and Prinz, W. 2001. "Perceptual Basis of Bimanual Coordination." *Nature* 414, 69–73.

10. Cole, J., Sacks, O., and Waterman, I. 2000. "On the Immunity Principle: A View from a Robot." *Trends in Cognitive Science* 4, 167.

Chapter 10

1. Toombs, K. 1993. *The Meaning of Illness*. Dordrecht: Kluwer.

2. Oliver, M. 1996. *Understanding Disability: From Theory to Practice*. London: Macmillan.

3. Merleau-Ponty 1962, p. 286.

4. Gravity is in one sense the big enemy for those with either tetraplegia or many other problems with mobility. Without gravity tethering them to a spot and a place, people would be far more easily able to move in their immediate environments. In the space shuttle, for instance, paraplegics would be at far less a disadvantage. I was not sure if it was coincidence that two of the men interviewed for the present volume had large pictures of a shuttle launch in their rooms.

5. Hill 2000, p. 120.

6. Reeve, C. 2002. *Nothing Is Impossible*. London: Century; New York: Random House, p. 12.

7. Ramachandran, V. S., and Blakesee, S. 1998. *Phantoms on the Brain*. New York: Morrow.

8. This may reflect the different part of the nervous system involved. Phantom limb perceptions after loss of a limb through a peripheral injury leave damaged nerve cells from that limb to send signals to the central nervous system of the catastrophe. In spinal cord injury, it is the central nervous system itself, the spinal cord, which is damaged and so may not be able to signal to the brain in quite the same way. This must, however, remain speculative.

9. Burke, W. 2002. "The Neural Basis of Charles Bonnet Hallucinations: A Hypothesis." *J. Neurol. Neurosurg. Psychiatry* 73, 535–541.

10. Ffytche, D. H., 2002. "Cortical Bricks and Mortar." *J. Neurol. Neurosurg. Psychiatry* 73, 472.

11. Ffytche, D. H., and Howard, R. J., 1999. "The Perceptual Consequences of Visual Loss: Positive Pathologies of Vision." *Brain* 122, 1247–1260.

12. Baron-Cohen, S., and Harrison, J. E. 1997. *Synaesthesia*. Oxford: Blackwell.

13. Cytowic, R. 2002. *Synesthesia: A Union of the Senses,* 2nd ed. Cambridge, MA: The MIT Press.

14. Botvinick, M., and Cohen, J. 1998. "Rubber Hands 'Feel' Touch that Eyes See." *Nature* 391, 756.

15. Driver, J., and Spence, C. 2000. "Multisensory Perception: Beyond Modularity and Convergence." *Curr. Biol.* 10, R731–735.

16. Pavani, F., Spence, C., and Driver, J. 2000, "Visual Capture of Touch: Out-of-Body Experiences with Rubber Gloves." *Psychol. Sci.* 11, 353–359.

17. Morris 1989.

18. In a recent article of advice on sex in *Forward,* the magazine of the SIA UK (2001, 45, 29–32), it was suggested that men have two sorts of erections after spinal cord injury. In incomplete injuries, normal "psychogenic" erections are possible and indeed usual. In those with complete upper cord injuries, reflex erections occur following direct stimulation in over 90 percent of people. To reproduce ejaculation is necessary, which requires an intact cord from the lower thoracic and below (unless artificial aids are used). During sex, people also have to be aware of the problems of urinary and faecal continence, and are advised to empty the bladder first and to keep a bag near.

19. There is some very preliminary evidence that in complete spinal cord injury there may be some residual sensation from the vagina in women through the vagus cranial nerve. Whipple, B., and Komisaruk, B. R. 2002. "Brain (PET) Responses to Vaginal-Cervical Self-stimulation in Women with Complete Spinal Cord Injury: Preliminary Findings. *J. Sex Marital Ther.* 26, 79–86.

20. Hockenberry, J. 1995. *Moving Violations.* New York: Hyperion.

21. Not for the first time I felt slightly ashamed of my gender.

22. Maybe women are attracted more by the whole person, who makes them laugh and whose company they enjoy, whereas men are more attracted physically and visually. Women are probably also more inclined to help others and support them than men. I am aware that all this is dangerous ground.

23. Morris 1989.

24. Phelps, J., Albo, M., Dunn, M., and Joseph, A. 2001. "Spinal Cord Injury and Sexuality in Married or Partnered Men: Activities, Function, Needs and Predictors of Sexual Adjustment." *Arch. Sex Behav.* 30, 591–602.

25. Stover, DeLisa, and Whiteneck 1995.

Chapter 11

1. The feeling of light touch as being painful is a well-known consequence of reorganization of pathways in the nervous system, probably at the level of his spinal cord injury, and is known as allodynia.

2. Brodal, A. 1973. "Self-observations and Neuroanatomical Considerations After a Stroke." *Brain* 96, 675–694.

3. Renoir, J. 1962. *Renoir My Father*, p. 404, quoted in Gearin-Tosh, M. 2002. *Living Proof*. London: Scribner, p. 239.

Chapter 12

1. Hill 2000.

2. James wrote a wonderful account of his learning to live with his new face, "Changing Faces." Originally published by Penguin, it is now obtainable from the charity he set up to help with the psychosocial support for those with facial visible difference and for wider education purposes, <www.changingfaces. demon.co.uk>. The ground-breaking work of this charity, led from the front by James, in support and social integration is a model for spinal cord injury, and indeed for many other impairments.

3. Picardie, R. 1998. *No Time to Die*, p. 103–104, quoted in Gearin-Tosh, M. 2002, p. 32.

Chapter 13

1. A few years ago, a young man with multiple leg fractures was being nursed on a bed with framed pulleys and splints in Southampton Hospital when one night he went missing. His friends had wheeled his bed through the hospital, lifted him into a van, and gone off to the pub.

2. Times have changed, one hopes.

3. Colin had the same problem with a return to the hospital, remember.

4. This began in Hampshire with "Project 81," the year, incidentally, of his accident. Three people living in a Cheshire Home, near Alton, went to the boss and asked how much it cost to keep them for a week. He had no idea, so they divided the number of people by the annual budget and came up with a figure, £400–500 per week. The three said that for £300 each they would go away, and that's how it started. It took them two or three years to negotiate it with Social Services, and then they left for their own lives in their own homes.

5. Stephen's doctorate was dedicated to Simon.

6. Nicholas Scott's daughter was involved in disability rights issues and so on the opposite side to her father. He became famous, subsequently, for being in a car that ran over someone in the street and did not stop. The driver of the car was never clear, though Scott's career was over.

7. Kubler-Ross, E. 1970. *On Death and Dying.* London: Tavistock.

Her original work was on the reactions of patients coping with the news that they had inoperable breast cancer. The book is astonishing in its apparent simplicity and in its humanity, and has justly become a classic for nurses and other paramedical staff. It is also amazing that she wrote it after she had been working with dying patients for only two and a half years. She is almost apologetic in "simply telling the stories of my patients who shared their agonies, their expectations and their frustrations with us."

She describes stages of reaction to the news of one's death. Initially there is a denial and isolation. This is followed, for instance, by anger and "bargaining," over pain control as the process continues. Often there may later be depression, both as a reaction to the news but also a preparation for the acceptance that most people appear to reach. Nearer the end she describes a perhaps unformed kind of hope, a hope which both sustains and allows people to find meaning in their lives and their suffering.

8. Melville-Brown, P. and Work Structuring Limited. 2000. *Evaluation of the Employers' Forum for Disability-Gateway Partnership Disability to Work Project.*

9. One consultant with DML was at a train company advising on the design of carriages. He was wandering through a set of new carriages when a man in a suit casually asked him his opinion of the toilet. The consultant savaged them and then proceeded to show how inadequate they were for a disabled person trying to use them at 100 miles per hour in a moving train. The be-suited man was the chairman of the train company about to sign a large check for the finished order. The check was not signed for some time, and the consultant made himself scarce.

10. One of them, Ian Waterman, featured in a previous book (Cole 1995).

11. Knowing London medical schools, it could have been a lot worse.

Chapter 14

1. I remembered Oliver Sacks' quotation from Auden: "Medicine is not a science; it is the intuitive art of letting nature heal herself."

2. Oliver, M. 1990. *The Politics of Disablement.* London: Macmillan, p. 63.

3. Zola, I. 1982. "Social and Cultural Disincentives to Independent Living." *Archives of Physical Medicine and Rehabilitation,* 63, p. 84.

4. Kubler-Ross 1970.

5. Oliver 1996, chapter 1.

6. Ibid.

7. Borstal was a name of fear in the UK. My parents once threatened to send me there unless I behaved.

8. Finkelstein, V. 1988. "Changes in Thinking About Disability." Unpublished ms pp. 4–5. Quoted in Oliver 1990, chapter 4.

9. He may have been the first wheelchair academic to be given his own personal chair.

10. Oliver 1996, chapter 7.

11. Ibid., p. 2.

12. Ibid.

13. Royal College of Physicians of London and The Prince of Wales' Advisory Group on Disability. 1992. *A Charter for Disabled People Using Hospitals.* London: The Royal College of Physicians.

14. Oliver 1990, p. 33ff.

15. Williams, G. H. 1991. "Disablement and the Ideological Crisis in Health Care." *Social Sci. Med.* 33, p. 517–524.

16. Oliver 1990, p. 35ff.

17. More recently, the World Health Organization has taken definitions of disability far further and proposed a complex classification based on natural and manmade products that can reduce disability, the environment, support and relationships, attitudes, services systems and policies, body functions, activities, and participation, which in turn include personal and social processes, interpersonal relationships and interactions, self care and work, community and social life, and mobility. This is a very comprehensive system, but also perhaps slightly cumbersome. <www3.who.int/icf.>

18. Oliver 1990, p. 65.

Chapter 15

1. Goodman, S. 1986. *Spirit of Stoke Mandeville: The Story of Sir Ludwig Guttmann.* London: Collins, p. 165.

2. Morris 1991, p. 10.

3. Crow, L. quoted in Shakespeare, T., 1992, p. 40. "A Response to Liz Crow." *Coalition,* September 1992.

4. French, S. 1993. Chapter 1.2, pp. 17–25 in Swain, J., Finkelstein, V., French, S., and Oliver, M. *Disabling Barriers—Enabling Environments.* London: Sage Publications.

5. Morris 1991, p. 10.

6. Hockenberry 1995, pp. 88–89.

7. There is a small herd of cattle at Chillingham in the North of England that has not been interfered with or artificially bred in over 800 years. The herd regulates itself and has fluctuated between thirty and eighty or so individuals over that time, with no new blood. When a mother gives birth, she leaves the

herd for a few days and then returns to introduce her newborn calf to the others. If they do not like it for whatever reason, it is killed.

8. There is a sense, however, in which the evolution of society and, with it, increasing healthiness, has had an effect. With improved health in western societies, so the ill health of a decreasing minority may have become more stigmatized. James Partridge, with the consequences of a facial burn, has suggested he might have been less socially disadvantaged a century ago when facial scars were more frequent than now. It was with a huge sense of freedom and relaxation that he walked along a street in India and no one gave him a second glance.

Chapter 17

1. One tetraplegic woman told me that when she was in the hospital her consultant used to talk to patients about sheep. Not as mad as it sounds. He reasoned that people would be asked their health by everyone day after day, and if there were a problem the staff would tell him. His job was to try to establish some human contact beyond the injury.

2. I remembered Nora Ellen Groce's beautiful book on deafness and sign language on Martha's Vineyard. There was a high prevalence of deafness on the island and so most people, hearing or not, spoke sign. Deafness was not a problem and the deaf fully integrated into society. Groce, N. E. 1985. *Everyone Here Spoke Sign Language: Hereditary Deafness on Martha's Vineyard.* Cambridge, MA: Harvard University.

3. Without control of the body and limited neck control one's balance is severely compromised. If this is a problem when first in a chair, on a horse or a boat it must be many times worse. Not only are you being thrown around unpredictably, but also one's relation with any fixed external frame of reference will constantly be changing, making calculations about where is up and your relation to the vertical very difficult. On a boat the only fixed point in relation to upright is the horizon, which is not always visible.

4. A friend told me of a friend of his who was tetraplegic. He had a car accident and was stuck in his car. When the rescue services arrived, he told them he had broken his neck. They panicked before he managed to make them understand that he had broken his neck years before and had just told them because he was unable to help himself out of the car.

Chapter 18

1. Gilman, S. L. 1999. *Making the Body Beautiful.* Princeton, NJ: Princeton University Press.

2. Hockenberry relates that his parents wonder if he has pushed himself further in life than he would otherwise to overcompensate for his paraplegia.

3. Hockenberry 1995, p. 256.

4. <www.changingfaces.co.uk>.

5. Goodman 1986, p. 116

6. Partridge 1990.

7. Murphy 1987, p. 178.

8. Hockenberry 1995, p. 78.

9. Oliver 1990, Chapter 5.

10. Pentland, W., Walker, J., Minnes, P., Tremblay, M., Brouwer, B., and Gould, M. 2002. "Women with Spinal Cord Injury and the Impact of Aging." *Spinal Cord* 40, 374–387.

11. Morris 1989, p. 22ff.

12. Goldstein, K. 1939. *The Organism: A Holistic Approach to Biology.* Boston: Beacon Press, p. 38.

13. Murphy 1987, p. 75.

14. Depraz, N. 2001. "The Husserlian Theory of Intersubjectivity as Alteriority." In Thompson, E. ed., *Between Ourselves. J. Conscious Stud.* 8, 5–7, 151–168. Thompson, E. 2001. "Empathy and Consciousness." In Thompson, E. ed., *Between Ourselves. J. Conscious. Stud.* 8, 5–7, 1–32.

15. Gallese, V. 2001. "The 'Shared Manifold' Hypothesis: From Mirror Neurons to Empathy." In Thompson, E., ed., "Between Ourselves." *J. Conscious. Stud.* 8, 5–7, 33–50.

16. Toombs, K. 2001. "The Role of Empathy in Clinical Practice." In Thompson, E. ed., "Between Ourselves." *J. Conscious. Stud.* 8, 5–7, 247–258.

17. One reason she did a Ph.D. was so that she would become Dr. Toombs, and might therefore be more influential with medical doctors.

18. Group Captain Sir Leonard Cheshire, VC, was a pilot from the Second World War who then dedicated his life to looking after disabled service personnel and those with incurable problems who needed full time care, by setting up homes and villages for them. I had always been given to believe that he was a saint; the idea that he locked people up and so prevented independent living never occurred to me as a child.

19. Brissenden, quoted in Oliver 1990, p. 173.

20. Oliver 1990, p. 57.

21. Murphy 1987, pp. 173–176.

22. Kannus, P., Niemi, S., Palvanen, M., and Parkkari, J. 2000. "Continuously Increasing Number and Incidence of Fall-induced, Fracture Associated, Spinal Cord Injuries in Elderly Persons. *Arch. Intern. Med.* 160, 2145–2149.

23. Nobunaga, A. I., Go, B. K., Karunas, R. B. 1999. "Recent Demographic and Injury Trends in People Served by the Model Spinal Cord Injury Care Systems. *Arch. Phys. Med. Rehabil.* 80, 1372–1382.

24. Zarb, G., and Oliver, M. 1993. *Ageing with Disability: What Do They Expect After All These Years?* London: University of Greenwich.

25. One is worried for some wheelchair athletes who stress their remaining joints in long-distance sports when they will need intact arms and shoulders for transfers and other movements as they age.

26. It is also far more difficult to have smears and mammography as a tetraplegic, so that screening is often not done.

27. McColl, M. A., Stirling, P., Walker, J., Corey, P., and Wilkins, R. 1999. "Expectations of Independence and Life Satisfaction Among Ageing Spinal Cord Injured Adults." *Disabil. Rehabil.* 21, 231–240.

28. Pentland et al. 2002.

29. McColl, M A. 2002. "A House of Cards: Women, Aging and Spinal Cord Injury." *Spinal Cord* 40, 371–373.

30. Pentland et al. 2002.

31. There is some evidence for the opposite, that as we all grow older then the effects of disability become less and that there is a levelling between those with an impairment and the able-bodied. Both have support, but the disadvantages may be uppermost.

32. Zarb and Oliver 1993, p. 37.

33. Pentland et al. 2002.

34. Pentland et al. 2002.

35. *Forward,* Magazine of the Spinal Injuries Association, April 2000, 36; p. 26–27. June 37; p. 28–29, October 2001; 39, p. 31–32.

36. Quoted in Oliver 1996.

37. Reeve, C. 2002. *Nothing Is Impossible.* New York: Random House/Century.

38. In discussing research, one should not forget those who have been influential in prevention. By altering rugby union laws, improving seat belts in cars, and pointing out the dangers of gymnastic trampettes, a number of spinal cord injuries have been averted in the UK. I have also skated over many issues, including a major one in the political processes involved in adequate funding for impaired people and the way of avoiding dependency while providing a minimum standard of care. The issues are tangential and just too huge for the present account.

39. Nietzsche, F. 2001. *The Gay Science.* Williams, B., ed. Cambridge: Cambridge University Press, p. 152.

40. Burchiel, K. L., and Yezierski, R. P., eds. 2002. *Spinal Cord Injury Pain: Assessment, Mechanisms, Management.* Published as vol. 23 of *Progress in Pain Research Management.* Seattle: International Association for the Study of Pain Press.

41. Pentland et al. 2002.

42. Gallagher, S. 2000. "Philosophical Conceptions of the Self: Implications for Cognitive Science." *Trends Cog. Sci.* 4, 14–21.

43. Shoemaker has talked of a sensory embodiment, a volitional embodiment— in which the body moves according to the person's commands, and a biological

embodiment—the autonomic functions such as sweating, blushing, and temperature control. Tetraplegics have a severely reduced sensory and volitional embodiment. In contrast, their biological embodiment is largely dysfunctional. Shoemaker, S. 1976. "Embodiment and Behavior." In Rorty, A., ed. *The Identities of Persons*. Berkeley: University of California Press, pp. 109–137. I am indebted to Professor Shaun Gallagher for bringing my attention to this work.

44. Merleau-Ponty 1962, p. 91.

45. Ibid., pp. 137–139, 146, 382–383.

46. Beckett 1938, p. 37.

47. Vasey 1999.

48. Ibid.

49. Ibid.

50. Swain, J., Finkelstein, V., French, S., and Oliver, M. 1993. *Disabling Environments–Enabling Environments*. London: Sage/Open University.

51. One of the first important realizations in the movement for independent living was that people with a given impairment could achieve more for themselves through joint collective action. The first such organization could have been the British Deaf Association, which was formed in 1890, followed by the National League for the Blind nine years later. It appears not to have been until after the Second World War that further organizations were founded, with the Disabled Drivers Association in 1949. Then there was another gap until the beginnings orthe modern time with the Disablement Income Group in 1965. Independent living schemes emerged in Berkeley in 1961. Originally, in the States, individuals such as Ed Roberts, with polio, and people born with impairments of one sort or another, took it up. Then it developed as a policy response, spread within the USA and Scandinavia, and was then taken up over by people with spinal cord injury. In the UK, those in Cheshire Homes were in the forefront of people who wanted to escape.

52. Reeve 2002, p. 105.

53. Merleau-Ponty 1981, pp. 435–437.

54. Mithen, S. 1996. *The Prehistory of the Mind*. London: Thames and Hudson.

55. This is homologous to software development rather than a simple increase in memory. Alan Turing, arguably the inventor of the modern computer, immediately saw that software flexibility, rather than memory capacity, would be crucial in computing.

56. Hockenberry 1995, p. 78.

57. Original Wittgenstein quotation from Monk, R. 1990. *Wittgenstein*. London: Jonathan Cape.

58. Murphy 1987, p. 179.

59. Hill 2000, p. 289.

60. Hockenberry 1995, p. 213.

61. Hockenberry 1995, p. 207.

References

Baron-Cohen, S. and Harrison, J. E. 1997. *Synaesthesia.* Oxford: Blackwell.

Beckett, S. 1957. *Murphy.* New York: Grove Press.

Beckett, S. 1958. *Happy Days.* New York: Grove Press.

Beckett, S. 1958. *The Unnamable.* New York: Grove Press.

Bell, C. 1833. *The Hand: Its Mechanism and Endowments as Evincing Design.* London: Pickering. Reprinted 1979 by The Pilgrims Press, Brentwood, Essex.

Botvinick, M. and Cohen, J. 1998. "Rubber Hands 'Feel' Touch That Eyes See." *Nature,* 391, 756.

Brodal, A. 1973. "Self-Observations and Neuroanatomical Considerations after a Stroke." *Brain* 96, 675–694.

Burchiel, K. L. and Yezierski, R. P., eds. 2002. "Spinal Cord Injury Pain: Assessment, Mechanisms, Management." *Progress in Pain Research and Management,* vol. 23, Seattle: International Association for the Study of Pain Press.

Burke, W. 2002. "The Neural Basis of Charles Bonnet Hallucinations: A Hypothesis." *J. Neurol. Neurosurg. Psychiatry* 73, 535–541.

Cole, J. 1995. *Pride and a Daily Marathon.* Cambridge, MA: The MIT Press.

Cole, J. D., Illis, L. S. and Sedgwick, E. M. 1987. "Pain Produced by Spinal Cord Stimulation in a Patient with Allodynia and Pseudotabes." *J. Neurol. Neurosurg. Psychiatry* 50, 1083–1084.

Cole, J. D., Illis, L. S. and Sedgwick, E. M. 1991. "Intractable Central Pain in Spinal Cord Injury Is not Relieved by Spinal Cord Stimulation." *Paraplegia* 29, 167–172.

Cole, J., Sacks, O. and Waterman, I. 2000. "On the Immunity Principle: A View From a Robot." *Trends Cog. Sci.* 4, 167.

Crow, L., quoted in Shakespeare, T., 1992. "A Response To Liz Crow," *Coalition,* p. 40.

Cytowic, R. 2002. *Synesthesia: A Union of the Senses,* second edition. Cambridge, MA: The MIT Press.

Damasio, A. 1999. *The Feeling of What Happens.* New York: Random House.

Depraz, N. 2001. "The Husserlian Theory of Intersubjectivity as Alterity." *J. Conscious. Stud.* 8, 169–178.

Driver, J. and Spence, C. 2000. "Multisensory Perception: Beyond Modularity and Convergence." *Curr. Biol.* 10, R731–735.

Ffytche, D. H. 2002. "Cortical Bricks and Mortar." *J. Neurol. Neurosurg. Psychiatry* 73, 472.

Ffytche, D. H. and Howard, R. J. 1999. "The Perceptual Consequences of Visual Loss: Positive Pathologies of Vision." *Brain* 122, 1247–1260.

Finkelstein, V. 1988. *Changes in Thinking About Disability,* unpublished ms pp. 4–5. Quoted in Oliver, M. 1990. *The Politics of Disablement.* London: Macmillan.

Forward, *Magazine of the Spinal Injuries Association,* April 2000, 36; pp. 26–27. June 37; pp. 28–29; October 2001 39, pp. 31–32.

Frank, A. W. 1991. *At the Will of the Body.* Boston: Houghton Mifflin.

French, S. 1993. In Swain, J., Finkelstein, V., French, S. and Oliver, M. *Disabling Barriers—Enabling Environments.* London: Sage Publications.

Frith, C. D., Blakemore, S.-J. and Wolpert, D. M. 2000. "Abnormalities in the Awareness and Control of Action." *Phil. Trans. R. Soc. B,* 355, 1771–1788.

Gallagher, S. 1986. "Lived Body and Environment." *Res. Phenomenol.* 16, 139–170.

Gallagher, S. 2000. "Philosophical Conceptions of the Self: Implications for Cognitive Science." *Trends Cog. Sci.* 4, 14–21.

Gallese, V. 2001. "The 'Shared Manifold' Hypothesis: From Mirror Neurons to Empathy." *J. Conscious. Stud.* 8:33–50.

Goodman, S. 1986. *Spirit of Stoke Mandeville: The Story of Sir Ludwig Guttmann.* London: Collins.

Gearin-Tosh, M. 2002. *Living Proof.* London, Scribner.

Gilman, S. L. 1999. *Making the Body Beautiful.* Princeton, NJ: Princeton University Press.

Goldstein, K. 1939. *The Organism: A Holistic Approach to Biology.* Boston: Beacon Press.

Groce, N. E. 1985. *Everyone Here Spoke Sign Language: Hereditary Deafness on Martha's Vineyard.* Cambridge, MA: Harvard University.

Hill, J. 2000. *Footprints in the Snow.* London: Macmillan.

Hobby, J., Taylor, P. N. and Esnouf, J. 2001. "Restoration of Tetraplegic Hand Function by Use of the Neurocontrol Freehand System." *J. Hand Surg.* 26B, 459–464.

Hockenberry, J. 1995. *Moving Violations.* New York: Hyperion.

Humphrey, N. 2002. *The Mind Made Flesh.* Oxford: Oxford University Press.

Kannus, P., Niemi, S., Palvanen, M. and Parkkari, J. 2000. "Continuously Increasing Number and Incidence of Fall-Induced, Fracture Associated, Spinal Cord Injuries in Elderly Persons." *Arch. Intern. Med.* 160, 2145–2149.

Kaspusinki, R. 2001. *The Shadow of the Sun: My African Life.* New York: Knopf, London: Allen Lane/Penguin Press.

Keith, M. W. et al. 1996. "Tendon Transfers and Functional Electrical Stimulation for Restoration of Hand Function in Spinal Cord Injury." *J. Hand Surg.* 21A, 89–99.

Kennedy, P., Rogers, B., Speer, S. and Frankel, H. 1999. "SCI and Attempted Suicide: A Retrospective Review." *Spinal Cord* 37, 847–852.

Kubler-Ross, E. 1970. *On Death and Dying.* London: Tavistock.

Leder, D. 1990. *The Absent Body.* Chicago: University of Chicago Press.

Ledoux, J. 1998. *The Emotional Brain.* New York: Simon and Schuster.

Manns, P. J. and Chad, K. E. 2001. "Components of Quality of Life for Persons with a Quadriplegic and Paraplegic Spinal Cord Injury." *Qual. Health Res.* 11, 795–811.

McColl, M. A. 2002. "A House of Cards: Women, Aging and Spinal Cord Injury." *Spinal Cord* 40, 371–373.

McColl, M. A., Stirling, P., Walker, J., Corey, P., Wilkins, R. 1999. "Expectations of Independence and Life Satisfaction among Ageing Spinal Cord Injured Adults." *Disabil. Rehabil.* 21, 231–40.

Mechsner, F., Kerzel, D., Knoblich, G. and Prinz, W. 2001. "Perceptual Basis of Bimanual Coordination." *Nature* 414, 69–73.

Melville-Brown, P. and Work Structuring Limited. 2000. *Evaluation of the Employers' Forum For Disability—Gateway Partnership Disability to Work Project.*

Merleau-Ponty, M. 1962. *The Phenomenology of Perception.* London: Routledge; Atlantic Highlands, NJ: The Humanities Press.

Merleau-Ponty, M. 1964. *The Primacy of Perception.* Illinois: Northwestern University Press.

Mithen, S. 1996. *The Prehistory of the Mind.* London: Thames and Hudson.

Monk, R. 1990. *Ludwig Wittgenstein.* London: Jonathan Cape.

Morris, J., ed. 1989. *Able Lives: Women's Experience of Paralysis.* London: The Women's Press.

Morris, J. 1991. *Pride against Prejudice: Transforming Attitudes to Disability.* London: The Women's Press.

Murphy, R. 1987. *The Body Silent.* New York: Henry Holt.

Nepomuceno, C., Fine, P., Richards, J. et al. 1979. "Pain in Patients with Spinal Cord Injury." *Arch. Phys. Med. Rehabil.* 60, 605–609.

Nietzsche, F. 2001. *The Gay Science.* Williams, B., ed. Cambridge: Cambridge University Press.

Nobunaga, A. I., Go, B. K., Karunas, R. B. 1999. "Recent Demographic and Injury Trends in People Served by the Model Spinal Cord Injury Care Systems." *Arch. Phys. Med. Rehabil.* 80, 1372–1382.

North, N. and O'Carroll, R. E. 2001. "Decision Making in Patients with Spinal Cord Damage: Afferent Feedback and the Somatic Marker Hypothesis." *Neuropsychologia* 39, 521–524.

O'Carroll, R., Ayling, R., O'Reilly, M. and North, N. 2003. "Alexithymia and Sense of Coherence in Patients with Total Spinal Cord Transection." *Psychosom. Med.* 65, 151–155.

Oliver, M. 1990. *The Politics of Disablement.* Macmillan: London.

Oliver, M. 1996. *Understanding Disability: From Theory to Practice.* London: Macmillan.

Partridge, J. 1990. *Changing Faces.* London: Penguin Press.

Pavani, F., Spence, C. and Driver, J. 2000. "Visual Capture of Touch: Out-of-Body Experiences with Rubber Gloves." *Psychol. Sci.* 11, 353–359.

Pentland, W., Walker, J., Minnes, P., Tremblay, M., Brouwer, B. and Gould, M. 2002. "Women with Spinal Cord Injury and the Impact of Aging." *Spinal Cord* 40, 374–387.

Phelps, J., Albo, M., Dunn, X. and Joseph, A. 2001. "Spinal Cord Injury and Sexuality in Married or Partnered Men: Activities, Function, Needs and Predictors of Sexual Adjustment." *Arch. Sex Behav.* 30, 591–602.

Picardie, R. 1998. *No Time To Die.* Quoted in Gearin-Tosh, M. 2002. *Living Proof.* London: Scribner.

Putzke, J. D. and Richards, J. S. 2000. "The Impact of Pain in Spinal Cord Injury: A Case Control Study." *Rehabil. Psychol.* 45, 386–401.

Ramachandran, V. S. and Blakesee, S. 1998. *Phantoms on the Brain.* New York: Morrow.

Reeve, C. 1998. *Still Me.* New York: Random House.

Reeve, C. 2002. *Nothing Is Impossible.* London: Century; New York: Random House.

Renoir, J. 1962. *Renoir My Father,* quoted in Gearin-Tosh, M. 2002. *Living Proof.* London: Scribner.

Rintala, D., Loubser, P., Castro, J. et al. 1998. "Chronic Pain in a Community-Based Sample of Men with Spinal Cord Injury: Prevalence, Severity and Relationship with Impairment, Disability, Handicap, and Subjective Well-Being." *Arch. Phys. Med. Rehabil.* 79, 604–614.

Royal College of Physicians of London and the Prince of Wales' Advisory Group on Disability. 1992. *A Charter for Disabled People Using Hospitals.* London: The Royal College of Physicians.

Rose, M., Robinson, J., Ells, J. and Cole, J. D. 1988. "Pain Following Spinal Cord Injury: Results from a Postal Survey." *Pain* 34, 101–102.

Rowe, D. 1983. *Depression. The Way Out of Your Prison.* London: Routledge.

Sacks, O. 1985. *The Man Who Mistook His Wife for a Hat.* London: Duckworth.

Scarry, E. 1985. *The Body in Pain.* Oxford: Oxford University Press.

Shoemaker, S. 1976. "Embodiment and Behavior." In Rorty, A., ed., *The Identities of Persons.* Berkeley: University of California Press.

Shoham, S., Halgren, E., Maynard, E. M. and Normann, R. A. 2001. "Motor-Cortical Activity in Tetraplegics." *Nature* 413, 793.

Stensman, R. 1985. "Severely Mobility-Disabled People Assess the Quality of Their Lives." *Scand. J. Rehabil. Med.* 17, 2, 87–99.

Stensman, R. 1994. "Adjustment to Traumatic Spinal Cord Injury. A Longitudinal Study of Self-Reported Quality of Life." *Paraplegia* 32, 416–22.

Stormer, S., Gerner, H. and Gruninger, W. 1997. "Chronic Pain/Dysaesthesia in Spinal Cord Injury Patients: Results of a Multicentre Study." *Spinal Cord* 35, 446–455.

Stover, S. L., Delisa, J. A. and Whiteneck, G. G. 1995. *Spinal Cord Injury. Clinical Outcomes from the Model Systems.* Gaithersburg, MD: Aspen Publishers.

Swain, J., Finkelstein, V., French, S. and Oliver, M. 1993. *Disabling Environments — Enabling Environments.* London: Sage/Open University.

Thompson, E. 2001. "Between Ourselves." *J. Conscious. Stud.* 8, 197–314.

Toombs, K. 1993. *The Meaning of Illness.* Dordrecht: Kluwer.

Toombs, K. 2001. "The Role of Empathy in Clinical Practice." *J. Conscious. Stud.* 8, 247–258.

Vasey, S. ed. 1999. *The Rough Guide to Managing Personal Assistants.* London: National Council For Independent Living.

Whipple, B. and Komisaruk, B. R. 2002. "Brain (PET) Responses to Vaginal-Cervical Self-Stimulation in Women with Complete Spinal Cord Injury: Preliminary Findings." *J. Sex Marital Ther.* 26, 79–86.

Whiteneck et al., quoted in Stover et al., 1995.

Williams, G. H. 1991. "Disablement and the Ideological Crisis in Health Care." *Social Sci. Med.* 33, 517–524.

Wittgenstein, L. 1980. *Remarks on the Philosophy of Psychology.* Oxford: Blackwell.

Zarb, G. and Oliver, M. 1993. *Ageing with Disability. What Do They Expect after All These Years?* London: University of Greenwich.

Zola, I. 1982. "Social and Cultural Disincentives to Independent Living." *Arch. Phys. Med. Rehabil.* 63, 84.

Index

Italics indicate those people whose narratives are featured within the text.